T0119737

Freelance Writing on Health, Food and Gardens

Freelance Writing on Health, Food and Gardens

Susie Kearley

**COMPASS
BOOKS**

Winchester, UK
Washington, USA

First published by Compass Books, 2014
Compass Books is an imprint of John Hunt Publishing Ltd., Laurel House, Station Approach,
Alresford, Hants, SO24 9JH, UK
office1@jhpbooks.net
www.johnhuntpublishing.com
www.compass-books.net

For distributor details and how to order please visit the 'Ordering' section on our website.

Text copyright: Susie Kearley 2013

ISBN: 978 1 78279 304 5

All rights reserved. Except for brief quotations in critical articles or reviews, no part of this book may be reproduced in any manner without prior written permission from the publishers.

The rights of Susie Kearley as author have been asserted in accordance with the Copyright, Designs and Patents Act 1988.

A CIP catalogue record for this book is available from the British Library.

Design: Lee Nash

Printed and bound by CPI Group (UK) Ltd, Croydon, CR0 4YY

We operate a distinctive and ethical publishing philosophy in all areas of our business, from our global network of authors to production and worldwide distribution.

CONTENTS

To my husband, Victor. Thank you for believing in me and supporting me, while I follow my dream.

Chapter 1

Introduction

So you want to write for the health, food and gardening markets? That's good news because there are lots of opportunities, although you'll need plenty of persistence and determination to break down doors and make those valuable contacts.

Health, food and gardening are intrinsically linked. Vegetable gardening, fresh food and recipes have an obvious connection, which in turn, is pretty closely related to health – because home-grown vegetables are the world's healthiest foods. It's easy to see how all three topics would suit some gardening magazines, but also, how some health and foodie magazines might be interested in gardening too.

It's not just magazines – there is an abundance of newspapers, online publications, and books dedicated to (or just interested in) these subjects, offering a multitude of opportunities across different media platforms to write for pleasure, for profit, and for the satisfaction it brings.

Selling articles on health, food and gardening, is what I've been doing since becoming a professional writer in 2011. This book explains how I achieved that goal, the approaches and techniques that worked for me, and it explains how to overcome some of the obstacles to achieving your goal as a published writer of health, food and gardening articles – as well as perhaps authoring a book or two!

But first, let me introduce myself. Today, I am a full-time freelance writer, but it hasn't always been that way. It was a huge step for me when I decided to go it alone in the middle of a recession!

I had the writing bug even as a small child – I dreamed of

writing children's adventure books. I was an avid reader, even before I went to school. I loved English and excelled at it. Then as I grew up, I wanted to become a horror novelist. This was a more serious aspiration – to be the next James Herbert.

The dream never transpired. Despite my enrolling on a writing correspondence course when I left school, and attempting to throw myself into it full-time, my parents had other ideas along more conventional employment lines. I spent all day filling out application forms for jobs instead – this was not the kind of writing career I had in mind!

After considerable failed attempts to get work during the 1990s recession, I enrolled on a two-year 'training' scheme, which turned out to be little more than legalised slavery. With a 3-hour commute each day, I was too exhausted to read, study, or write very much. My writing ambitions were going nowhere.

Two years on, I got a part-time job in a shop which gave me more time to dedicate to my craft. That was when I achieved my first success with an article published in *The Lady*. However, after three years of trying to make it as a part-time writer, one published article failed to hit the spot. It just felt like too little, too late.

By 1994 I'd done a year's service in the shop and submitted a failed management application. I thought *there must be more to life than this*, and enrolled on a psychology degree at the local university. It sounded like a plausible alternative, with good career prospects (or so I thought).

I started writing again in my spare time and had some interest from Hodder Headlines in a book I was working on, but after some to-ing and fro-ing, they rejected it, and I didn't have the confidence to try any other publishers, thinking my work must be seriously flawed.

After completing my degree, to my dismay, I found that my aspirations for a career in psychology were on a par with aspirations for a career as a writer. I just couldn't get a break. I tried to get a voluntary position in social services or addiction counselling – but apparently other volunteer applicants had more experience than me! I couldn't give my services away for free.

I applied for a place on a postgraduate journalism course and went up to London for the interview. I took a test, failed (I've never spelt liaison wrongly since!) and came home miserable and disillusioned. Was I destined to live with my parents forever?

A year later, I met my husband in a dead-end office job. Then I retrained in marketing at the age of 25. A ten-year career in marketing ensued (thank goodness!), helped in part, by my wonderful husband who built up my confidence, making a huge difference to my career prospects.

Marketing communications enabled me to unleash some of my creativity and hone my writing skills. I wrote promotional literature and learnt graphic design. Even a period working for a self-confessed bully couldn't get me down. I kept bouncing back – much to her annoyance!

During a slow period at work I wrote e-books and sold them online. Then I qualified in nutrition in 2007 and practised as a part-time therapist for a full year until the onset of the 2008 recession, which killed the fledgling business almost instantly.

That year I also started a new marketing job. I enjoyed it overall, but my superiors didn't like my clear and concise style of writing – they wanted literature full of corporate jargon, industry buzz words, and puff. This really wasn't my world at all.

By 2009, I'd started to doubt my own writing ability. Had I spent 20 years in a delusional state, thinking I was good at it?

I took voluntary redundancy a year and a half later, followed by a couple of short term contracts. Then I had a spell working in a very small business, which made me realise just how good my writing skills really were, compared to some of their seasoned professionals in the field of journalism.

The company used freelance journalists with impeccable credentials to write brochures and PR material for their clients, but as I saw their work pass across my desk I was horrified. It was dreadful. There were meaningless sentences, dreadful grammar, terrible spelling, and whole words missing in the text. There was a total lack of care and attention, and worse still, due to a lack of proofreading prior to my appointment, the company had gone ahead and printed their contributions without any editing. The office was littered with brochures full of errors. I pointed out a huge blooper in the first line of a promotional brochure, and the boss quietly organised reprints – with corrections.

The experience provided a surge of confidence in my own ability, confirming what I'd really known all along. I was damned good at writing (and proofreading actually!). I thought 'if these journalists can succeed in the publishing industry I can do it standing on my head!' The standard of work in the small company, combined with a boss who was suffering from an anger management problem, gave me good reason to part company with the firm six weeks later. But the experience in that small business had served its purpose, transformed my outlook and given me renewed drive to try writing again.

Driven by renewed vigour and a strong belief in my own writing ability, I attempted to launch myself as a freelance writer. I worked long hours, with sheer grit and determination, until I succeeded.

In the end, it was simply a return to my roots – writing was the only thing I'd ever been really good at. My husband had faith in me which helped a lot. I had no way of knowing whether I would succeed, but I gave it my best shot and importantly, although I wasn't bringing in much income, in the early months, my husband supported me 100%.

Within months I had a regular column with the local newspaper and started to get work with magazines securing commissions to write about gardening, military history, food, nutrition and travel. I found my greatest selling point was my nutrition qualification and diversity of knowledge about natural health.

I looked for inspiration everywhere, and started writing about gardens, wildlife, ponds, and vegetable plots for gardening magazines. I became something of a nuisance pitching so many nutrition ideas to magazines that they couldn't ignore me. Some gave me work while others probably blocked my emails.

As my portfolio of published work grew and grew, Dad started offering me copies of magazines that he'd come across – thinking I could write for them. Mum started buying copies of the magazines publishing my work. The two people most sceptical about my writing ambitions, were silenced by my success… well, nearly silenced. I get the impression Dad still thinks I'm too young to be a writer. I'm in my 40s!

Various elderly relatives were keen to appear in nostalgic magazines and told me their true stories of war-time nursing and military service. Dad cooperated with an article about his years working on the railways.

For the first 6 months, I was still keeping my options open and attending marketing interviews, unsure whether I could make the writing pay as a full-time occupation. Work was slow and the pay was erratic. But as time passed, the work continued to trickle in, and within about 9 months, I had the confidence to dedicate 100% of my time to writing. I have never looked back and now I am incredibly busy.

I found myself frequently working on the three topics of food, health and gardening – all linked to my fascination with health and nutrition.

In my first year, I earned a very modest living writing about food and nutrition. I created recipes for health magazines, gardening and smallholding publications, and started to see early successes writing for general interest magazines.

It takes a huge amount of tenacity and determination to succeed in this marketplace but I put everything into it, and now I'm working with some big names including the BBC. It's hugely competitive and many freelance writers supplement their income with other work. I don't. I am a full-time freelance writer, and I specialise in subjects relating to health, food and gardening. Would I be making a better living if I were running workshops too as many freelance writers do? Possibly. I haven't written it off, but at the moment I focus on writing, and on the photography that illustrates my work. Do I earn as much as I did as a marketing manager? Not at the time of writing, but my income is growing steadily and I'm optimistic. I earn a living and I enjoy it, which is more important.

I joined the local writers' group and the photographic society this year to boost my social life and better my skills. My writing journey is an experience that I'm thoroughly enjoying, and I hope this book can help to give you the confidence that you need to realise your aspirations, and follow your dreams.

Exercise

Write down your ambitions. What do you hope to achieve in:

- six months?
- one year?
- three years?

Now make a list of food, health and gardening topics that you'd like to cover. Consider which magazines might be interested in your work and use this as a guide, or a mini plan, to help get you started in these markets.

Chapter 2

Writing health articles for magazines and newspapers

The number of health magazines on the market is vast. In Britain they include *Top Sante, What Doctors Don't Tell You, Feel Good You, Healthy Magazine*, and *Women's Health*. Irish titles include *Easy Health*; Australian titles include *Natural Health*, and *Vegetarian Magazine*; and in the USA, the leading titles include *Shape*, and *Prevention*, to name just a few.

When I started writing on health and nutrition, I had the benefit of 8 years' study and was a qualified nutritionist. This opened doors, enabling me to develop my workload quite quickly in this competitive area – but it's not essential.

That's not to say you don't need some level of expertise. Health is too important to pretend you know what you're talking about if you don't. Journalists do make silly mistakes on health pages from time to time, and for those of us who have appropriate training and know what we're talking about, their errors stand out like a sore thumb. Worse, if they're dishing out bad advice, it's downright irresponsible.

I did get the opportunity to write health pages from one magazine after getting their attention by pointing out their errors. I told them that omega 3 is not an antioxidant but a pro-oxidant (they were confused so I sent them papers on it). They said 'not carrots but carotenoids!' so I explained that carrots are loaded with carotenoids making the statement a nonsense (the clue is in the name). They said it's a myth that carrots help you see in the dark – but actually they contain betacarotene and vitamin A, which help to prevent night blindness. So it's not a myth.

I had nothing to lose – they'd been ignoring my emails for a year. Quite remarkably, the approached worked in my favour for that particular publication. However, when I tried the same approach with another publication whose writers and editors clearly didn't understand the difference between bacterial infections and fungal infections, I was met with a stony silence.

If you're not an expert in a field of health, then stick to interviewing the experts and reciting the latest research findings in a way that is relevant to your target publication. Incorrect information in this area can have serious consequences, so do double check everything. Provide information, not advice, and suggest people check with their doctor before embarking on a new health regime.

When you are writing for the health market, you have a responsibility to the reader and their health. A number of high-profile authors have been taken to court by people who didn't get on with their dietary regime – among the most famous was Dr Atkins, the creator of the Atkins Diet. Dr Atkins probably had insurance for this eventuality but I'm guessing you don't. Insurance is covered in Chapter 21.

Generally I tread very carefully when I'm writing about health. Most of the publications I work for have a very fleeting interest in cutting edge approaches to natural health, mainly because they often challenge the conventional wisdom of modern healthcare and conflict with our western culture and modern lifestyles.

Radical claims about the benefits of natural healthcare are often considered to be too extreme, unless the publication itself is radical. It's a very rare editor indeed who actually believes that good nutrition and detoxification have the combined power to cure cancer!

It's also worth being aware that scientific studies do offer conflicting results, and it can be helpful to look at a range of studies to get the balance of opinion. Nothing is absolute, but there is one thing that scientists agree on: most people in Western society don't eat enough fruit and vegetables.

Where the science is conflicting or inconclusive, I try to give a balanced perspective in my writing, because I feel it's important to not mislead people. For example, one study conducted a few years ago, concluded that a little alcohol every day increases your life expectancy. Notably, the study was conducted amongst men, and the biggest improvement was seen with red wine consumption which helps to reduce the risk of heart disease because of its high levels of antioxidants. These benefits have not been shown among women, but other studies have shown that every glass of alcohol consumed increases a woman's risk of breast cancer. I wasn't about to start recommending ladies drink alcohol every day with statistics like that. But I did see an article in a woman's magazine that did just that, completely ignoring that the study was conducted on men and presumably written by someone who didn't do their homework.

Make sure you know your subject inside out before giving out health advice.

Taboo subjects

As you continue to study health, you'll find, if you haven't already, that there are certain taboo subjects where many magazines are concerned. It's less of an issue for some newspapers but I've found that many magazines won't touch anything about serious toxicity or bowel problems and they are very reluctant to speak about cancer. Some publications dependent on advertising say that advertisers will not have their adverts placed beside an article on cancer. They don't want the association – and for that reason the editors are not interested in running stories about how food and lifestyle choices may help to prevent cancer.

Toxicity is another taboo subject. While detoxification regimes are all the rage, stories of serious toxicity are usually too controversial for mainstream publishers. Where I did have a great story about a woman suffering from toxicity symptoms, I found a spiritual angle and sold it to a spiritual magazine.

Articles on bowel problems are in low demand because no one likes to talk about the bowel – or apparently read about it. Although you might be lucky if you find a suitably tasteful angle on the subject of something quite common like IBS. It took me two years' working in health journalism before I managed to secure a commission on the topic of bowel complaints.

Other taboo subjects include some of the controversy surrounding dairy products. Milk is widely considered to be a health food in western culture, yet some experts claim that it is detrimental to health. This is a widely debated area, with some of the more controversial ideas beautifully summed up in T Colin Campbell's book, *The China Study*.

However I've found that as a health writer working mostly in conservative markets, there's only so far you can push ideas that fly in the face of western culture and conventional wisdom. It is acceptable to write about dairy alternatives for those people with allergies, and those interested in the different choices available – but start discussing controversial ideas that challenge cultural norms, and you might find yourself hitting a brick wall.

Of course, you're free to try pitching anything, but in my experience these areas can be troublesome.

Diversity of opportunities

In health writing, there are many different types of practitioner – reflexologist, naturopath, kinesiologist, reiki practitioner, massage therapist, nutritionist, yoga instructor, Pilate's teacher, osteopath, hypnotist, positive thinking guru, homeopath, herbalist, acupuncturist, spiritual healer, chiropractor, dietician… the list goes on.

You may be not be convinced by the virtues of them all – especially at the prices some of them charge – but they do all offer potential as interview candidates and they provide a wide diversity of different perspectives on natural health, from which you can draw article ideas. Any one of these disciplines could provide the foundation for a health article, but it's more likely to sell if you include case studies of real people who have benefited from the therapy together with good pictures.

Interviewing health practitioners

Although I have qualified in nutrition myself, occasionally I need to interview other health practitioners for my articles. I find the direct approach works best, so I just walk in and ask! I've done that with the owner of our local crystal healing shop, and when I needed an interview with an herbalist, I contacted a practitioner who had been recommended to me. Offering to plug their latest book or website is always a nice gesture if you're asking them to share their time and expertise with you.

Many health articles are led by case studies of individuals – some of whom have seen miraculous results. Finding someone who's been cured of a horrible disease by switching to a raw vegan diet might be tricky, but there are people around with stories to tell, and if you keep your ears open, you might be surprised with the number of useful contacts you make. When the case study is the lead story, editors usually want a story that hasn't been covered in the press before. So while you might be able to track down someone who has cured her cancer with a raw vegan diet, if her story is plastered all over the internet then you either need to come up with a different angle, a new approach, or to offer it as part of a bigger feature on a raw lifestyle.

When someone's miraculous story is the main focus of the article, they often expect to be paid for their cooperation. Some real life magazines recognise this and offer a separate fee for the interviewee. This is ideal. However, many magazines don't, so if your interviewee wants paying, and you have to split the fee, it might not be worth your while doing it. One way to work out whether to accept a job like this is working out your hourly rate for doing it, and then decide whether it's enough to warrant committing the time to the project, which you might otherwise spend on other tasks.

Another fantastic resource for finding interview subjects is social media. I find Facebook invaluable for finding short case studies to accompany articles – even as I write this book, I have, in the last week, found three people among my Facebook friends, willing to contribute to stories as short case studies.

Interviews can be really enjoyable and come together quite quickly. They are often straightforward. You don't have to go digging around doing research. The interviewee tells you what you need to know and all you have to do is get it down in a way that reads well, flows nicely, and meets the word count. I have done all manner of interviews with health practitioners, pastors, and performers.

Occasionally I've gone out into the local community to find a suitable case study for an article. On one occasion I was tasked with interviewing a lady with arthritis who found alternative medicine provided some relief. My Facebook requests failed, my contacts weren't coming up with anything. So in the end, I went to the local coffee morning where I found a lady who met my criteria in minutes and she agreed to help. It was a short piece and the interview only took about five minutes. Then we went outside, took a few photographs, and within weeks it was in a woman's weekly magazine. So when you get really stuck, a local coffee morning is a great place to go, to find a wide range of people, all looking for someone to talk to.

Writing the perfect pitch

So you're just getting ready to pitch a few ideas to the editor of a health magazine, but he or she has never heard of you. Why should they consider giving you the opportunity?

The best way of securing a commission, is to ensure that you have three key things: a strong hook, qualifications or experience in the subject, and a track record of published material to your name.

Let's break this down. A strong hook can be a special date, a link to a television show, or something current in the news. You need to show the editor why he or she should publish the article, and why they should publish it imminently (remembering that some publications have long lead times).

One good source of 'hooks' on health topics, is Science Daily. I've signed up to email alerts with www.sciencedaily.com to have all the latest research delivered straight to my email inbox every morning. This is a great source of newsy material on which you can elaborate, according to your specialism or your pool of contacts.

Why should the editor assign you to write the article? It's important to demonstrate a thorough knowledge of your subject matter, whether that's self-hypnosis, nutrition, or crystal healing. Either outline your qualifications and experience, or identify your expert interviewees and provide their credentials. If you have contacts and resources that the publication doesn't, this also works in your favour.

Finally, being able to demonstrate that you have published work to your name is important to some editors, and a link to your website for examples is usually sufficient. If you don't have examples of published work, an editor may ask to see the finished article 'on spec', with a view to accepting it if it's suitably well written.

Some editors prefer samples of your work to be attached by email, and they'll usually tell you if that's what they want.

Wider markets for health-related articles

As you can see from the list of practitioners, health topics start to diverge into sports activities, and there are opportunities to write about health in sports magazines, walking magazines, newspapers, online, and general interest magazines. But it doesn't end there. Religious publications, and even business publications are interested in health – I've sold articles on stress and nutrition to a variety of business publications too.

All over the western world, people are tired, burnt out, stressed, and not coping. Everyone's worried about their health, and they should be, because the incidences of serious disease are rising at an alarming rate. It seems like almost everyone's medicated on something. Readers almost everywhere are interested in health.

Spiritual publications with an interest in health also exist – most notably in the UK, they include *Soul and Spirit*, and *Spirit and Destiny*, and they are interested in health and beauty, horoscopes, psychic powers and spells. They carry true life stories of women who have had remarkable healing experiences with a spiritual twist. They might also include tales on developing your sixth sense, or divine weight loss.

Other spiritual publications with a focus on health and healing, include *Caduceus, Kindred Spirit,* and *Prediction*. They all cover a myriad of unusual alternative therapies and spiritual healing techniques. Sometimes they'll touch on nutrition and run more conventional health articles too.

Readers' Slots

Don't forget the opportunities provided by readers' slots in real life magazines like *Take a Break, That's Life, Pick Me Up, Love It, Chat, Real People* and *Full House*. They are all looking for health stories, detailing dramatic recovery from a dreadful disease or a tragic accident.

If you outline your own health story as a regular reader and submit it, they will contact you if they like it. Then they will interview you and write it up themselves. That's fine. You still get paid, and some of them pay very well.

Funnily enough, unlike some more traditional magazines, the true life sector is not averse to hearing about dramatic and impossible-sounding natural health claims. If there's someone willing to be interviewed and photographed about their dramatic recovery from a nasty disease, using only laughter therapy and green smoothies, then that's good enough for them.

You can also target readers' slots as a professional journalist, on behalf of someone else who is willing to sell their story. If they accept your query, then you write it up. It's quite likely that the editors will change your copy considerably before it goes to print, but they usually read it back to the interviewee first.

Read read read

The other thing I'd strongly recommend to anyone interested in writing for the health market is to read, read and read some more. There is such diversity of opinion, and conflicting research, both within the scientific world, medical profession, and across the spectrum of other therapies, that you can't really write about health with any authority until you've heard a good number of the arguments and theories, and have started to form an educated opinion on what really does constitute optimal nutrition, a healthy lifestyle and what works in terms of natural approaches to healthcare.

There is some cutting edge reading available in the health sector and among my personal favourites are *The China Study* by T Colin Campbell, and *Detoxify or Die* by Sherry Rogers. Patrick Holford's *Optimum Nutrition Bible* is a great place to start if you're interested in writing about nutrition. But I'm not convinced about his emphasis on nutrient supplementation – partly because in my wider reading, there is evidence that high quantities of selected nutrients over extended periods can do more harm than good.

The reading and learning you undertake enables you to make these sorts of educated judgements for yourself. So follow the latest research, be open minded, and constantly reevaluate what you think you know.

Exercise

Write down all your areas of expertise, and all your contacts in the health industry, then outline some article ideas that you'd like to sell, and identify some target publications for these articles. Study the target publications to see whether your ideas are a good fit, and if you still think they are (and your interviewees are willing to cooperate), send off your pitch to the relevant editor and see what comes back. Good luck!

Chapter 3

Writing for the food and cookery press

I write about food and nutrition for health publications, women's magazines, gardening magazines, recipe magazines, and even religious publications. If food is your passion, there's a huge market for articles on the subject.

The obvious examples in the UK are magazines like *BBC Olive, Delicious, BBC Good Food, The Healthy Food Guide,* and *Vegetarian Magazine.* In the USA there is even a magazine dedicated to tea, simply called *Tea Magazine.*

Just like writing for the gardening market, you don't need to be a professional cook to sell recipes – but it helps if you have a basic ability to create a distinctive recipe of your own and take a good picture of it. Traditional recipes with a twist usually go down well.

That said, not all food writing requires recipes. You might be more interested in the travel side – visiting restaurants, sampling cultural cuisine from different countries, or going on a wine tasting tour. Reviewing authentic Italian cuisine might be more up your street, or perhaps at the most extreme end of food journalism, you could join an Amazonian tribe to discuss the delights and health credentials of raw beetles. Yum!

But let's get back to recipes for the moment. As part of my nutrition training, I created my own dishes with healthier alternatives to the ingredients listed in more traditional recipes. I would invariably use healthy fats instead of butter. I'd never include sugar, and I'd use whole-grain ingredients when the original recipe required white flour. Sometimes I'd use less fat and other times I'd want to achieve a low carbohydrate dish, so I'd cut right down on grains or use seeds instead.

This opened up a market for me to sell healthy recipes as

alternatives to the unhealthy foods that most people cook and eat.

Decent photographs of the finished recipe are, of course, a prerequisite. It must look like something you'd be prepared to pay good money for in a restaurant.

There are all sorts of specialist markets within food writing and because some of them are quite niche, they might be easier to break into than general magazines. Take for example, *Get Fresh* magazine, a publication produced by the Fresh Network, primarily about the health benefits of the raw vegan diet. That's an extreme diet to write about and it's essential to know the rules of raw vegan dining. Raw vegans often use dehydrators to slowly warm their food without breaking down the nutrients. Nothing is heated above 48°C. They are also very interested in health issues, in fresh local produce, and in growing your own. It's another good example of how closely related food, health and gardening writing can become. However, niche publications like this are rarely inundated with specialist writers on these topics. Another example of a niche publication in this sector is *Vegetarian Magazine*. Opportunities in the vegetarian market might include articles on different varieties of cheese, or even a day out to Cheddar Gorge to see cheese-making in action.

Any kind of food production – chocolate factory visits or brewery tours for example – might appeal to magazines that cover food topics. They don't need to be magazines focusing exclusively on food either. Numerous general interest magazines include recipes and food-inspired travel. Look to see what the foodie publications, and others dabbling in this area are publishing now. Get a feel for what their readers are interested in, and offer similar but different ideas.

One publication to be aware of when you're having a slow time, is *Take a Break's My Favourite Recipes*, which offers readers £25 for every published recipe. It's very easy to submit your recipe, and because they use so many, it's pretty easy to get published as long as you send a tasty looking photo of your finished dish.

Food interviews

One of my most recent interviews with a restauranteur was a commission from the local newspaper to visit a local restaurant and sort out the copy for their advertorial. The conversation went a bit like this.

"Hello, it's Susie Kearley calling on behalf of the Bucks Herald."

"Who?"

"Susie from The Bucks Herald."

Silence.

I continued, "The local newspaper? They told me you contacted them wanting to place an advertorial – and that you wanted someone to write it for you?"

More silence, then, "Oh yes."

"Can I come to see you to discuss it?"

Date was fixed. I arrived on time. We met and sat down.

"OK. What do you want covered in this advertorial?"

"I don't know."

"OK. What makes you different from any other restaurant in the area?"

"I don't know."

Now, I won't bore you with the entire transcript, but you can see it was hard work. I ended up dragging his 'Unique Selling Proposition' out of him (that's marketing jargon for what you offer that no one else does). It turned out that his little restaurant offered a wonderful experience – a fusion of old and new with traditional dishes available alongside modern novelty dishes. It is all beautifully presented and served on banana leaves, just as it is in the temples of India, with music from Slumdog Millionaire playing in the background. The completed transcript came out like this, and the client was delighted:

Duo Chefs – Fusion Indian Cuisine
Step into a world where you can experience the best of South Indian culture, combined with culinary excellence, and a friendly smile.

The newly named 'Duo Chefs' in Chinnor fuses ancient tradition with a modern approach to dining. Most dishes are served on banana leaves, just as they are in the Temples of Southern India. The innovative menu, however, may come as a surprise!

"The restaurant is our passion and our dream," say partners Abdul and Abdul, who have recently joined the owner, Mr Ahmed, at the restaurant, "We aim to provide a unique experience and pride ourselves in creating new and innovative dishes to meet people's individual needs. We cater for all tastes and dietary requirements, and if you want something special, it's no trouble – just ask."

Alongside traditional dishes, you can expect the unexpected at Duo Chefs. The menu offers a range of unique and unusual meals, carefully created by your hosts. Examples include 'Scallops & Squid Chilly Fry' for fish lovers, 'Lamb Coconut & Chillies' and 'Dark Tamarind & Honey' – these are favourites with customers.

But why stop at the menu? These friendly chefs will cook anything you request, exactly the way you like it – options are limited only by your imagination!

Don't forget to leave space for pudding. Duo chefs serve fresh mango, or you can enjoy a traditional Indian dessert called Gulaf Jamun – warm doughnuts served in a warm syrup. It's a satisfying way to finish the evening if you have a sweet tooth.

Abdul and Abdul pride themselves on the restaurant's friendly ambience. Your enjoyment is their top priority. Dine in a relaxing environment, with background music from the Oscar winning film, 'Slumdog Millionaire'.

Both chefs have 18 years' experience working in restaurants around the South East. They cater for birthday parties, outdoor events, and wedding parties. Innovative dishes, aromatic spices, and fresh high-quality ingredients keep their customers coming back again and again.

I thought that was quite reasonable for a restauranteur who didn't know what his USP was! If you're working with a chef covering the recent opening of a new restaurant, hopefully he'll be a bit more forthcoming. But if he isn't, you need to really probe. Find out what makes his customers keep coming back. Find out what inspired his business model. Get him to tell you about the menu, the music, the ambience – and if you have time and budget allows, why not experience it all for yourself!

Another recent submission was an article on growing onions which I prepared for a gardening magazine. It provided a detailed breakdown of onions' health credentials, explained how they can help to prevent disease, and included a couple of recipes which contained a high proportion of onions. I tested these recipes and took pictures before submitting the article. You can see how an article like this crosses all three sectors – health, food and gardening.

Writing recipes for magazines is clearly a very different ballgame to writing advertorials for small businesses. You've created your recipe, but you need to write the rest of the blurb to go with it. What makes it great? Just follow the style of the magazine. Most of my own recipe articles cover the health benefits of the recipe over and above the usual junk food version of the same thing. I always use wholegrain flour, and the world's healthiest ingredients, but your talent might be in making the world's lightest and fluffiest cakes, so that's what you need to put across in your complementary blurb – not forgetting top class photographs.

Writing the perfect pitch

Writing the perfect pitch for food magazines follows the same principles as in gardening writing. Your 'hook' might be Pancake Day, Easter, Valentine's Day or something linked to recent news. Or it might be that a publication has an upcoming issue on

Scandinavia and you're perfectly placed to write about Scandinavian cuisine. Perhaps you've lived there and have a few contacts in the trade, or you are about to go on holiday there and can do reviews of some of their top eating houses.

Do be aware that parts of the food market may be driven by editorial themes, worked out months in advance, so it's worth checking with the editor of your target publication if they have monthly themes set for the year ahead. Sometimes the themes might be healthy salads, or chocolate indulgence, while at other times, like when they're scheduling the Christmas edition, they'll be looking for something very specific to the time of year, like unusual canapés for your Christmas party.

It may be helpful when you're producing recipes, if you have a background and qualifications in cooking. However it's not essential and if you can produce good photographs of a recipe that looks really tasty, then that could be sufficient to secure your place in your chosen magazine.

Wider markets for food-related articles

Everyone loves food. You'll find food-related articles in numerous publications, from newspapers, to women's magazines – even the travel sector covers the best restaurants in exotic locations, visits to vineyards, and sampling French cheese.

It can be easy to sell the same recipe ideas to different markets too. For example, I have sold salad dishes to gardening magazines, smallholding magazines, women's magazines, religious magazines, and health magazines.

All you need is a different angle with each approach. When selling food topics to religious magazines you need an angle to do with God or religion – so, you might sell something to do with Lent – perhaps a recipe for a chocolate alternative for those people giving up chocolate.

When you sell a recipe to a gardening magazine, it can be helpful to have a gardening link, such as harvesting your own salads – or the different types of tomatoes that you might grow on your vegetable plot, along with a commentary about their virtues and how difficult or easy they are to grow.

If you're selling food articles to women's magazines, then winning story lines might include losing weight, summer barbecues, or how salads can help to keep your skin beautiful – often accompanied by a couple of tasty recipes.

When you're targeting health magazines you need a clear health benefit – such as how certain foods can help to reduce the pain of arthritis, or help protect against cardiovascular disease.

Don't overlook the professional sector in food – small business magazines might be interested in the lady who's built up a business in her kitchen making fancy cakes... and I bet she'd be willing to tell you all about it!

The key is to take your foodie subject, and tailor it to any magazine that you intend to target – whether that's in the business market where you might need to demonstrate that this food helps you concentrate, or keeps you alert during meetings; or whether it's the children's market where you're simply demonstrating the fun of cooking.

Once you start to think how you can target foodie articles into the most unlikely locations, you might be surprised at just how successful you are.

Exercise

Make a list of the publications that you'd like to target with your food and cookery articles. Analyse copies of the magazines and jot down some ideas of topics you could sell. Do you have the time, patience and equipment to get top class photographs? Or someone on hand to do it for you? If not, avoid the photography-led magazines until you are better equipped to meet their needs, and focus on the topics you can cover for other publications – those for whom a quick snapshot on a compact camera is fine.

Chapter 4

You don't need to know about gardening to write for gardening magazines – but it helps!

It's true. My earliest commissions came from writing about the health benefits of fruit and vegetables for a gardening magazine. I didn't know much about gardening or growing vegetables at that time, but I did know how the nutrients in vegetables help to combat disease.

As I browsed the pages of the gardening magazines in the newsagent, I realised that you don't need to know about gardening to write for gardening magazines. Even astrologists write for gardening magazines – detailing the optimal planting patterns according to the cycles of the moon!

There are many gardening publications available in the UK including *The Edible Garden, Your Garden, The English Garden, Garden News, Permaculture, BBC Gardeners' World,* and numerous others. There are also smallholder magazines, professional journals for landscapists and groundsmen, and many more titles on the fringe of gardening journalism. In the USA there is *Organic Gardening magazine,* and *Country Gardens;* and in Australia, *ABC Gardening* is a market leader.

Obviously, if you're serious about writing for these markets on a regular basis, it helps enormously to know about gardening, to be qualified in horticulture, and have the appropriate experience and credentials to back you up as an authority on the topic. If you do have all these virtues, then there are lots of opportunities in this market, and all you need to do, is study the market and come up with some winning stories, secure the commissions, and then write them up in an engaging manner.

You can cover composting, organic gardening, pest control,

raised beds, lawn care, floral borders, garden schemes and garden design. You could even write a humorous piece about the cute little mouse in the compost heap that your partner doesn't think is so cute, for any publication that likes a touch of wit! The list could go on. Just use your imagination.

For those people wanting to break into the gardening market without much knowledge of gardening, you need to demonstrate your worth by coming up with new and interesting topics where you can show some level of expertise – or have good pictures and valuable interviewees to hand.

When I started researching Druidry for an article in a spiritual magazine, I came across a website about the Druid garden, which after conducting interviews with Druids in the UK and learning a little more about Druidry myself, inspired me to write about a Druid's approach to gardening. Druids you see, are strong proponents of the natural world, and oppose the damage caused by pesticides and intensive farming. Obviously, growing your own vegetables is much more sustainable and can be done without the use of pesticides by a skilled organic gardener who has knowledge of some natural pest repellents and how to use them.

Druids are interested in saving seeds – because so many varieties of seed have vanished due to intensive farming practices, and because of big business monopolies on seed availability (in the USA). Some intensive farming practices are bad for the environment, and for local ecology. I've written articles on a Druid's approach to gardening, which included some unusual ideas, such as spiritual gardens and playing music to your plants, alongside the more conventional organic methods of growing your own produce.

Other subjects that could be of interest to gardening magazines are bee-related topics such as how to have a bee-friendly garden, coverage of the National Trust's 'save the bees' campaign, or an interview with a beekeeper. There's been a dramatic decline in the bee population in the UK, and around the world, which is thought to be due to pesticide use. At the time of writing, governments arguably don't seem to be taking the threat as seriously as perhaps they should. The declining bee population could have catastrophic consequences for our food chain, as it prevents plants being pollinated so they fail to bear fruit. This is all of interest to gardeners.

The plight of the declining bee population opens up debates about the toxicity of pesticides, bee-friendly plants, and beekeeping stories. These issues also cross over into the health market, providing the germs of ideas for health publications too.

Think widely about gardening and your ideas can open doors, enabling you to report on all sorts of things that you wouldn't necessarily associate with gardening magazines. There are opportunities for interviews, reports on stately homes and gardens, opportunities to cover flower shows, and to interview community groups about their community growing projects.

Don't forget the opportunities within the smallholding magazines and professional landscaping magazines. Both gardening and smallholding magazines run recipes from time to time.

Gardening interviews

In my experience getting interviewees for gardening articles is really easy – but it might be helped by the fact that many of my gardening articles have been on the topic of stately homes where the PR people, keen for the publicity, have put me in touch with their head gardeners. It doesn't have to be the head gardener however – beekeepers and volunteers make great interview subjects too. I'm not fussy!

I also do on-the-spot interviews when the opportunity presents itself, by having a chat with a gardener and then asking if it's OK to quote them in a hypothetical article (if I manage to get a commission for it). When I visit a stately home, I rarely have a commission for an article in advance, but getting a few comments from the gardener can help to secure the commission. Then if necessary, I'll have a longer chat with the gardener over the phone.

Sometimes I write visitor experience articles and find that this brief conversation with the gardener provides an interesting and valuable additional perspective for a gardening magazine. If you use informal chats in this way, keep it short and simple so you can remember it accurately. Write down what was said as soon as you can.

Sometimes, when I visit these locations, people are doing talks and I just happen to be passing by. It turns out that what they are saying is really interesting and it makes it into one of my articles.

I do take great care to accurately reflect the meaning of what they said, even if the words are different, and if in doubt, I get in touch, email them the relevant extract from the article, and ask them to check it. People are usually very helpful.

For a more detailed interview piece, a formal interview, recorded either on a notepad or Dictaphone is a much better arrangement, which provides a reliable transcript of what was said.

While I do generally think it's a good idea to check your final draft with your interviewee, I did once wish I'd done things rather differently. I'd interviewed a volunteer gardener extensively over the telephone. He was involved in a National Trust garden restoration project, and had actually told me that he was the head gardener. It transpired that he wasn't – he was a volunteer. This didn't matter. But it mattered that I had a two-day deadline. I sent him the article, which I felt reflected our telephone conversation accurately, asking for him to approve it or make any minor modifications that he felt were necessary. Imagine my reaction when I received the returned manuscript, completely rewritten. He took out all the quote marks, so it was no longer an interview piece. What he returned was completely unsuitable for the magazine.

I tried to contact him to reach some kind of compromise – and to find out whether he was genuinely no longer willing to be quoted or whether he just didn't understand – but he stopped communicating with me altogether, ignored my emails and wouldn't answer the phone.

I got in touch with their press office to try to rectify the situation. That was when this 'head gardener', turned out to be a volunteer. They had originally said they'd get 'someone suitable' to call me back, and when he called, I asked if he was the head gardener, he said 'yes' and I had no reason to disbelieve him!

Anyway, titles didn't matter. This guy knew enough about the project, but with my deadline looming, if he wasn't going to speak to me to work out a compromise, I needed to start again with another interviewee.

However, fortunately at the 11th hour, the press office got a senior gardener to have a chat with him and it all came together. They called me back, saying the original piece was fine. The deadline was met, photographs submitted – job done. That was the tightest deadline I've ever nearly missed!

After that, I developed a reluctance to offer my completed article for approval to any interviewees – although it doesn't take much to persuade me otherwise. Fortunately I haven't had any similar experiences since.

Writing the perfect pitch

So you're ready to pitch to the editor of a gardening magazine. You need a strong hook, qualifications or experience in your subject, and a published work to show your background and professionalism as a writer.

A special date in the gardeners' calendar could provide a strong hook, as could a relevant television show, or something current in the news.

To provide a good example of a strong 'hook', my husband and I went on holiday to Avebury Henge in 2011, and by pure coincidence, The Manor Reborn with Penelope Keith had been filming there just days before. We were among the first to see the Victorian kitchen garden restored to its former glory.

I returned from the holiday, and immediately pitched an idea to cover the story of the restoration project to run in parallel with the television show. I received the commission and it was one of the shortest deadlines I've ever had.

Don't miss opportunities like that – when you're in the right place at the right time, make sure you've got your camera with you, take loads of photographs so that you've got some good ones among them, and don't be afraid to phone up and interview the head gardener, or another significant figure.

I've interviewed head gardeners and beekeepers in the past – most people have something interesting to say if you ask open-ended questions.

So now we've established that you need a strong hook, but what about qualifications or experience? Well it's important to demonstrate a thorough knowledge of your subject matter – whether that's in the history of landscape design, astrology, nutrition, ecology, wildlife, or something else. If you can't demonstrate that you're an expert, then the alternative is to have access to a suitable expert who you can offer as a willing inter-viewee.

If you plan to write about Druid gardening, you will need to demonstrate that you have contacts who are Druids, and that they are willing to be interviewed and photographed. If you plan to cover gardening at a stately home, then you will almost certainly, need to demonstrate that you have excellent photographs available to accompany the article, as well as suitable interview candidates.

Dig out relevant published work where possible to demon-strate your experience as a professional published writer.

Wider markets for garden-related articles

It's worth mentioning here, that you shouldn't limit your gardening writing to gardening magazines, because many general interest publications are interested in gardening articles too – especially if you're a horticulturalist. Look at women's magazines, home and garden magazines, lifestyle magazines, local newspapers, national newspapers, and some of the magazines that are published alongside them. Think widely about who could possibly be interested in your subject. How about bird watching magazines on the topic of a bird-friendly garden? Try to think outside the box – there are many opportunities in this field.

Women's magazines might be interested in articles that show how gardening helps to keep you fit and trim. Business magazines might be interested in the story of how an entrepreneur set up and grew a successful horticulture business – whether that's a garden centre, plant nursery, landscaping business, or an online shop for garden tools.

A health magazine might be interested in vegetable gardening from the perspective of the plant nutrients and their benefits to health, combined with the benefits of exercise from gardening activities. They are equally likely to be interested in the health benefits of garden herbs.

Religious magazines might be interested in how getting one-to-one with nature in the garden brings them closer to God – with the case study of someone who's benefited from this activity in their spiritual life.

Children's magazines might be interested in how things grow – for that matter, so might popular science magazines such as *How it Works*.

Spiritual magazines might be interested in something about mythical garden spirits and pagan approaches to gardening. Okay – that's starting to sound a bit off the wall, but it does demonstrate the widening scope for writing for all sorts of publications, once you start thinking outside the box.

Exercise

Write down all your areas of expertise that might be of interest to a gardening magazine. Then create a list of feature ideas, linked to these areas of expertise. Choose the best one, and practise writing your pitch. What's the hook? Is there anyone you would hope to interview for the piece? What samples of your work might impress the editor?

Chapter 5

Writing about health, food, and gardening opens doors to new opportunities

I quickly discovered that one story is rarely just 'one story'. Every piece I work on seems to open doors to new markets. Back in 2011, among my very first commissions, was a piece about the restoration of Hughenden Manor's walled kitchen garden. It had been transformed from a derelict plot of overgrown land, to a pretty kitchen garden, maintained by volunteers, and used as an educational resource for local school children and the local blind club.

I went to visit the walled garden and chatted with one of the volunteers working on the plots. He was friendly and happy to show me around and tell me all about it. I asked his permission to quote him and took his photo, but I didn't have a commission to write it up yet. I took more photos of the garden and the plots and returned to my writing desk, hoping to gain an assignment to write about the renovation project. I quickly secured a commission with a gardening magazine.

When I returned to Hughenden Estate later that month to take more photographs, I joined a guided tour of the house. Victorian Prime Minister Benjamin Disraeli lived there from 1848, until his death in 1881. He was a writer and journalist who launched a newspaper called The Representative, with his business partner, John Murray. They had ambitions to get rich in business, but it was a disastrous venture which failed within 6 months, incurring huge debts for both investors.

To help pay off some of his debts, Disraeli wrote a novel – a thinly disguised account of his newspaper publishing experiences. The novel was entitled Vivien Grey and it became a best-seller – it was a cynical portrayal of London's high society and they all bought a copy to see if they were in it.

I thought Disraeli's story was an interesting tale so I sold an article about his life and his first novel to a small British literary magazine.

I didn't stop there. While researching Disraeli's writing online, I found out that his ghost reportedly haunts the manor grounds. They've had paranormal investigators in doing research and everything! So I contacted the National Trust press office and they put me in touch with a medium who said she'd experienced Disraeli's presence in the drawing room. I wrote up her story for a spiritual publication.

Then I did a lengthier piece on the Hughenden Ghost for a paranormal magazine. To complete this article, I returned to the site, did the ghost walk, and took photographs of all parts of the house that had reportedly been privy to Disraeli's ghost. The staff thought I was mad.

Some months later, I wrote a piece on the life of Benjamin Disraeli for an historical publication, and took pictures of the house and grounds to accompany the article.

Wanting to maximise on the opportunity, I produced an article on the Manor's war-time history for a military history magazine and interviewed a veteran from the 1940s when the manor was run as a top secret bomb-mapping base for Bomber Command, just a few miles up the road.

I also wrote a travel piece on the visitor experience today, taking in a combination of garden delights, history, walks and tearooms; and then I returned to cover the Manor's annual 1940s weekend for a nostalgic publication.

Most recently, I have covered Hughenden Manor for a US interiors magazine, covering the gothic architecture, Disraeli's dramatic 'budget' interiors, and the Victorian artefacts displayed at Hughenden today. Queen Victoria visited the Manor in 1877, which turned out to be a bit of a selling point. I also worked Hughenden's ghost into a short story for the quick fiction market.

You might be wondering what all this has to do with writing for the health, food and gardening markets? It's a simple example of how one topic can lead to a multitude of stories. What started out as a simple piece for a gardening publication, quickly became a source of ideas for numerous other publications too. There are opportunities all around you, if only you can open your mind to see them.

I've diversified widely on health and food topics too. I started with a basic theme: how garden produce helps cure disease, or *The Healing Power of your Plot*. This story has the potential to cover so many different ailments and topics within the field of health and nutrition, that it can be written many different ways. I sold the concept to two different gardening magazines and a Scottish lifestyle publication, using different examples and different scientific studies in each, to demonstrate the same points – fruit and vegetables reduce your risk of heart disease, cancer and stroke... among other things.

Then I extended this idea, to write a piece for a management magazine on brain foods – a concept that I later sold to a motoring magazine and a couple of regional magazines. Each time, they were written up with different examples, quoting different studies – but they all discussed the same broad concept that healthy foods increase your brain power and concentration.

Before I knew it, I was writing for a science magazine too, covering 'The Science of Detoxification', 'How the Liver Works' and 'The Science of Baking'.

Just let your mind wander and you'll never be short of ideas. Ideas open doors. If you start writing about salads, you might find yourself writing about summer salads, superfood salads, and nutty salads... all slightly different angles on a theme, many with wide appeal across different markets.

Exercise

Start with a topic that you intend to write up for a health, food or gardening publication and write it down. Then list all the other possible angles on this basic concept, which might appeal to a wider audience.

How can you rework this idea for a new market?

What other opportunities are there to elaborate on the theme?

How can you use the same concept in a different context?

List all the different angles you can think of.

Chapter 6

Researching the markets

When you're looking for inspiration, it can help to look through magazines and see what they are publishing. Try to become familiar with their approach, their readership, and their style. All these things can be important when you're pitching feature ideas to them.

Researching the market will always provide insight and usually, a degree of inspiration. It's also worth looking at the writers' trade books for information on what different magazines are looking for. The Writers' and Artists' Yearbook (UK), Writers Market (USA), and the Australian Writer's Marketplace, will give you a feel for what different publications are interested in.

Health

Natural Health (UK) magazine's latest edition covers:

- Have you got Candida?
- Healthy weight – spice up your diet
- Aromatherapy explained
- Inner self – use your vulnerability
- Mediterranean recipes
- Personalities: the people pleaser
- California dreaming: looking good in the sunshine
- Yoga healing
- Boost your sexual power
- Natural cures for ADHD

So based on these stories, they might be interested in an article on natural cures for arthritis, how to get beautiful skin, a new therapy, or healthy recipes. Perhaps you have a personal true life story that could form part of a health article for this publication.

Feel Good You magazine, published by *Woman and Home*, covers the following topics in a recent edition:

- 20 minute workout
- How to sleep better
- Vitamins and minerals to stop you getting ill
- A three-day superfood diet
- How to have energy all day
- Finding time for the things you love
- Three steps to smoother skin
- Growing in confidence

You can see there are opportunities to touch on weight loss, fitness and toning, how nutritional supplements can benefit your health, and topics around beauty.

Food

BBC Good Food Magazine's latest issue contains features on:

- New summer flavours
- Simple suppers
- Healthy recipes
- Relaxed entertaining
- Fresh ideas for strawberries
- Summer barbecues
- Create your own spice blends
- Learn to make jam
- Special recipes for Fathers' Day

The edition contains 85 recipes, so there is plenty of scope for freelancers with new recipe ideas.

The latest edition of *Delicious* magazine focuses on the following topics:

- Foodswap: a food sharing community
- Raymond Blanc's foolproof chocolate fondant
- A summertime menu, bursting with the aromatic flavours
- Go meat-free for a week
- Shortcut suppers for quick and tasty meals
- How to be a better cook
- New ideas for chicken, meat and fish

Are you inspired by these features in the food markets? How about winter stews, vegetarian delights, double chocolate heaven, or fish delicacies?

Gardening

In a recent edition of *Garden Answers*, they ran the following features:

- Create a perfect patio
- Plan now for colour that lasts
- Climbing plants
- Meet the professional gardeners
- How to enjoy tulips
- Summer planting
- Pest control
- Water gardens
- Give nesting birds a hand
- Growing vegetables
- Try some exotic crops
- Watering your plants

Perhaps you could write something on helping the wildlife in your garden? Interview a professional gardener? Or cover a water garden near you?

Garden News magazine was running the following features this month:

- Chelsea Flower Show review
- Boost borders with bedding
- Testing long-handed trowels
- Trying new plants
- Growing for showing
- Tales from the Allotment
- Secrets of a garden designer
- Professor Stefan Buczacki recommends his favourite fruit collection
- How to make your garden a safer place for wildlife
- A look at remarkable weather
- Interview with head gardener at Floors Castle Gardens, Scotland

So this magazine publishes interviews with gardeners from stately homes and castles. Perhaps you could speak to the gardener at your local stately home, or what about covering your local flower show?

For those wanting to sell to US gardening magazines, this site might prove useful:

www.freelancewriting.com/guidelines/pages/Gardening.

Whatever your specialism, you can find inspiration in the pages of magazines, and hone your ideas to meet their requirements. Always check online to see if they have contributor guidelines or drop them an email and ask. These guidelines can help you frame your pitch. It means you're more likely to be successful than by sending a cold pitch without having read their guidelines first.

Exercise

Identify which magazines you'd most like to work for, and drop them an email asking for their contributor guidelines. Then, when you receive them, compose a query email for each, double check that it meets their guidelines and send it off. Good luck!

Chapter 7

Meet other successful writers in this field of work

Amanda Hamilton, health writer

Amanda Hamilton is a nutrition expert, broadcaster, writer and consultant whose passion for her subject coupled with her professional and engaging approach have made her one of the media's favourite and most respected businesswomen.

In television she is an established presenter, with a back catalogue of programming for the BBC, ITV and satellite channels that spans a decade. She has published three books, the most recent of which, *Eat, Fast, Slim* has just been released.

She is a registered nutritionist with BANT, a senior associate of the Royal Society of Medicine and a member of the Guild of Health Writers. She is in great demand as a consultant and guest speaker across a diverse range of sectors. Her background in business (in the technology sector), international-level sport and media has created a unique profile in the well-being industry that has led to her being labeled as 'one of the health industry's most effective communicators.'

Since its launch in 2011, Amanda Hamilton's weight loss diet has won the support of many medical doctors and has recently been nominated for an industry award. She has also worked as an advisor with the Scottish Government's Curriculum for Excellence panel on food and health. She has a number of charitable roles and has recently been signed up to host the Mary Portas 'Living and Giving' fashion show.

In her spare time Amanda is a keen skier, ad-hoc runner and devoted yogi. She trained in yoga during a sabbatical spent in an Indian ashram. She is also an ex-international badminton player. Amanda is 38, married, and she splits her time between

Edinburgh and London, living with her husband and children, ranging in age from age 3 to 18.

Qualifications

- BA Communications, Napier University.

- Dip Nutritional Therapy, Registered Nutritionist with BANT (British Association of Nutritional Therapy).

Q: What captured your imagination first: a love of writing, broadcasting, or a passion for natural health?

A: My passion for natural health came first – it just so happened that my strengths lay in communications rather than in research or academia. It took many years to find a way to put the subject at the core of my working life. My career in TV was really diverse before I made a conscious decision to move away from general presenting to being only an "expert". I don't think for a second that my career path has been the most sensible in terms of stability or consistency – but, I've been driven by a deep, abiding interest in health, which in its own way, is priceless.

Q: What was your first piece of published work?

A: At the age of 17 I got a summer job editing the youth section of a regional newspaper, so I started young! I had a decade-long relationship with that publication in the end, including being sent off to East Germany to report on a fascist uprising amongst disenfranchised skinheads while I was at university. Reporting and editing for that newspaper led naturally to reporting for TV news, which then opened up the opportunity for a career in television. It all starts with having a passion for finding out the story behind the story – my medium just happened to be one which has led to a certain amount of recognition.

Q: I see you have a new book out. What inspired you to write the new title?

A: It has been a consolidation of more than ten years' work with fasting so I really wanted to do it. I had to wait until my youngest child was old enough for me to take it on – I'd written a book with a baby in tow before and it's not something I wanted to do again! As it happened, I got the commission for this latest book just after my son started nursery – good timing!

Q: What have been the highlights of your health writing career?

A: I am most proud of my new book 'Eat, Fast, Slim'. I found a publisher who was happy for me to write with my real 'voice' – I shared many personal stories that are woven through the book. I think it is unusual in the health market. I also had a lot of fun doing it – there is humour in there too!

Q: What have been the greatest challenges you've faced as a health writer?

A: Turning ideas into reality is always the greatest challenge. Good ideas are ten a penny, making them happen is the tough bit! I pitched the latest book many times before it got commissioned – and now it's a best-seller and is being released in many countries. If you really believe in something, be tenacious.

Q: What advice would you give to anyone wanting to become a writer in the health sector?

A: Have a passion for it. You should be the type of person that lives and breathes the subject. Or, you could simply have a desire to seek the deeper story behind the headlines. Either could lead to success and satisfaction.

Q: Is there anything else you'd like to share?

A: Nothing happens overnight. I believe it is entirely true that you create your own success.

Amanda's new book 'Eat, Fast, Slim' is available from Amazon and high street retailers, price £8.99 or visit www.amandahamilton.co.uk for links to her online weight loss club, health retreats and blogs.

Jackie Lynch, health writer

Jackie Lynch BA Hons, Dip ION, mBANT, is a fully-qualified nutritional therapist. She is accredited by the Complementary & Natural Healthcare Council, a government-sponsored registration body for complementary healthcare practitioners. She is also a registered member of the British Association for Applied Nutrition and Nutritional Therapy and the NHS Directory of Complementary and Alternative Practitioners.

Her advice features regularly in a wide range of national newspapers and magazines, including *The Mail on Sunday, Sunday Mirror, Natural Health Magazine, Zest, Marie-Claire* and *Vogue*. She has also appeared as a guest expert on the *Let's Talk Living* magazine programme on the *Body in Balance* channel.

Alongside her writing activities, Jackie works in clinical practice, with people suffering from a variety of chronic health conditions. She works with those who are keen to take a preventative approach to their healthcare or improve their general well-being. She has an extensive knowledge of the impact of nutrition on health and well-being, and is proud to be the Chairman of the Board of Governors at the Institute for Optimum Nutrition.

Q. How did you first get into writing for the health markets?
A. Many nutritional therapists (70-80%) have to look for ways to supplement their income because it's not easy to make a full-time living out of clinical work alone. Some do teaching, run workshops, or try their hand at writing to develop other income streams. Others work part-time in conventional jobs and practice nutritional therapy as a sideline. Very few therapists make a full-time living out of clinical practice alone. When I started my training in 2006, I didn't anticipate completing it during a recession, but by the time I qualified in 2010, the recession had set in, making starting a new business an even greater challenge.

Nutritional therapists are self regulated – there is no statutory regulation, which means we are restricted to private practice and this has a cost implication for potential clients. Dieticians are used by the NHS for nutritional advice because they are part of mainstream healthcare, but nutritionists can't currently work directly for the NHS, which limits our opportunities for clinical practice. I work in clinical practice three days a week. If I did it five days a week, I think it would be too intense in any case – the emotional investment and focus required for each consultation can be quite draining.

In 2010, the recession had hit demand for nutritional therapy quite badly, so I decided to try writing for a second income, and for the publicity it would generate. My first opportunity to be published came quite unexpectedly when I was practising nutritional therapy at a yoga clinic in Kensington. The PR lady thought it was quite novel to have a nutritional therapist at the clinic and asked me to contribute some expert comments in the media, and write a blog to boost the profile of the clinic. I wasn't getting paid for my writing at this point – I was just doing it for the publicity. I didn't hit a paying market until January 2012.

My main break came when I made some personal contacts with editors. I hired a PR person for six months and she kept me really busy with writing work. I did something for *Zest* and a number of other publications, answering questions and providing quotes for articles written by other journalists. The word count was really strict and it helped me to focus on getting things clear and concise. This was really useful training, providing the skills to fulfil my writing ambitions over the months that followed.

Q. How did you make the leap from PR into journalism?

A. I was keen to move to something written by me, rather than contributing to someone else's work. I met a lady at a yoga holiday retreat, and she turned out to be the deputy editor of the review section in the *Mail on Sunday*. I stayed in touch with her and submitted a few ideas, but the paper didn't take me up on any of them.

Then one day, I got a commission – a small piece about the world of nutritional therapy. It was my first paying piece of journalistic work. From there I gained the confidence to pitch more targeted ideas and have recently featured in a double page spread in the *Mail on Sunday*. The article was a nutritional analysis of takeaway food. I learnt a few things in the process: it made me realise that successful freelance journalism is all about having the idea in the first place. Think creatively about what you can do, and then try to match it to what the market wants. Writing about McDonalds wasn't the first thing I thought of as a nutritional therapist wanting to get into journalism, but it reflected the real society that we live in – and importantly, it met editorial requirements. Surprisingly some of McDonalds' food wasn't as bad as I thought! Now, I always think, what's in it for the person who'll be reading this?

Q. What are the greatest challenges you've faced in your writing career?

A. Getting a good brief can be a challenge. With that first piece of work, the brief wasn't as clear as it might have been. The other big challenge for me has been the word count limitations. I'd say to anyone thinking of working in freelance writing, don't be overindulgent and try to get everything in. The editors come back with amendments, and I've even found that sometimes they change the angle of the article completely!

That, of course, presents another challenge, the dilemma of having your name put to something that's changed dramatically – and perhaps you're no longer comfortable with it. It's quite a balancing act, meeting editorial requirements, without compromising your experience and integrity as a professional in your field. Be brave and stick to your guns.

Q. What advice would you give to someone wanting to break into freelance writing for the health market?

A. It helps to study each publication so that you can get the feeling and prose accurate. I've also learned that you've got to be very proactive in going out and getting the work. And don't undersell yourself.

I sent a couple of ideas to *Inspired Health* magazine. They replied saying they'd like me to write the articles, but added that they don't usually pay. Over the last couple of years, I've gained confidence and learnt that my expertise is worth something. So I said 'no' to writing the article for free, and offered to write it for a fee. I set out my terms and my payment conditions. The editor went very quiet and I thought he'd lost interest, but then a couple of months later, completely out of the blue, he emailed me with a commission – a paid commission! I've learnt that editors won't pay you if you keep offering to write for free. Once you've got expertise and a portfolio of work, it's important not to do everything for free – or as writers, we will never make a living!

I've also found that meeting people helps. I've had doors opened by making connections on LinkedIn, not just in writing but in other lines of work too. There's no point being shy, or being scared to ask. Once you have an introduction it opens doors.

Freelance writing really requires you to be proactive. I didn't make any money at it for a while but it gave me good discipline and helped me turn things around quickly. If you're struggling to get started, and don't have the PR contacts, then an alternative approach is offering to contribute to your local newspaper.

Although freelance writing is difficult to break into, it's worth sticking with it because it's so rewarding to see yourself in print. I like writing. I've learnt a lot.

Jackie's website is: www.well-well-well.co.uk

Nick Baines, food writer

Nick Baines is a food and travel writer based in the UK. He contributes to *The Times, The Guardian* and *The Independent* amongst other national and international media; both online and in print. He is a certified barbeque judge for The Kansas City Barbeque Society, and a judge on The Great Taste Awards, and The World Cheese Awards. In 2012 he judged the Kate Whiteman Award for Work on Food & Travel for The Guild of Food Writers

Awards. Nick has also appeared on the *Good Food Channel* programme, *Market Kitchen*.

Nick sometimes moonlights as a copywriter, generating content for websites, catalogues and advertising.

Q. What captured your imagination first: a love of writing or a passion for food?

A. Writing came before the food. I used to snowboard a lot and lived in Austria for a couple of winters. My friends all turned pro whilst I never really cut the mustard so I began writing about their progress for snowboard magazines. My first piece of published work was a report on a British snowboard competition for a magazine called *SnowboardUK*.

It was a few years later before food grew to be an important interest for me. My first food and travel related piece was for *The Bournemouth Echo*, a local newspaper. It was about the end of the shooting season and it included a recipe that used pigeon breast.

Q. How did you first break into writing for the food market?

A. My writing for snowboard magazines led me to a full-time position as an editorial assistant at *SnowboardUK*. One Christmas, whilst at the magazine, my dad bought me a cookbook, which at the time was quite an odd present – it was *Jamie's Italy*. For one reason or another I cooked a pork chop dish from the book for my family one night when they were visiting and everyone was really impressed, which felt good and to be honest, I'd found it very therapeutic spending the afternoon going out for the ingredients and taking my time preparing the food. It was shortly after this meal that I was made redundant in advance of the snowboard magazine folding. I'd grown tired of the snowboard industry to be honest and was increasingly becoming obsessed with food, so I focused my freelance pitches on food and travel stories. I started writing regular food features and recipes for my local paper and things gradually progressed from there.

Q. What inspires your articles?

A. Much of my food writing has a travel focus. Travelling is my biggest inspiration and eating all kinds of regional foods is always what drives me. I'm an inquisitive and enthusiastic eater. I do have a few stock dishes up my sleeve, but I don't write a lot of recipes.

Q. *I see you have a blog – do you find that regular blogging is beneficial to your career?*

A. My blog has been fun and gave me an outlet for ideas. It's a good way to keep writing and stay on point, but in recent times it has become more of a portfolio rather than carrying its own content as I've just been too busy.

Q. *What have been the highlights of your food writing career?*

A. An article I wrote for *The Independent* on the future of eating insects was referenced in a United Nations Food & Agriculture report, which I was kind of chuffed about. Other than that, I am always just happy to be able to travel as much as possible with the excuse that it is work, or less convincingly, 'research'.

Q. *What have been the greatest challenges you've faced as a food writer?*

A. Getting regular work. It's incredibly tough to get regular work and living from month to month is sometimes a bit tough. I supplement my food and travel writing with copywriting and creating content for brands as well as the odd stint behind a bar. Writing is rarely a lucrative career choice and I often have times where I question whether it was a good idea. Year on year I have slowly reduced the amount of supplementary work I have had to do to earn a living, but to be honest, I sometimes like the variation. The whole reason I think I like writing is the variety, working across subjects and adapting to current trends and ideas. I don't think I really suit a 9-5.

Q. *What advice would you give to anyone wanting to become a writer in the food sector?*

A. Don't expect to be able to make a living from it to start with. Even some of the writers I look up to and respect have told me recently that it has been several years since some of them have made a decent living from it. But it's not all doom and gloom. If you're happy to be flexible and perhaps supplement your work with something else, it can be very fun and rewarding.

Do your research before you pitch. I spend many hours each week keeping up to date with relevant news stories and reading the features in papers and magazines to keep up with what they are publishing. You don't want to pitch a story on edible flowers to *The Times* in June, only to have the editor reply telling you they ran a story on edible flowers back in February.

Don't bombard editors with too many ideas at once, and try to keep your pitches short and to the point. Your editor should be able to get the story in a few lines, not several paragraphs. But don't be afraid to chase them up if you haven't had a response within a week. I have had stories commissioned from just a gentle nudge asking if they have had time to consider the pitch I sent last week.

When you have a story idea, ask yourself why this story is relevant today, or the period you are pitching it for. Why should an editor run your story in this week's issue and not next week's, or next month's, or at all. The hook is the most important thing to help you get your feature commissioned. Sometimes your hook can be something from the news stream that isn't even food related.

Quote your sources, it often adds relevance and authority and can help immensely in a pitch.

Nick's Blog is www.lostinthelarder.com
You can follow him on Twitter at www.twitter.com/@nlbaines

Sue Ashworth, food writer

Sue is a freelance food journalist, recipe writer, advertorial and feature writer for the web and magazines. She also works in radio broadcasting and as a food stylist. She is a consultant to well-known food companies and PR agencies, working on high profile accounts.

Her work varies from managing, developing and executing major projects through to food styling for packaging and editorial work. She enjoys radio work and has written and presented many pieces. Her specialities lie within the health, slimming and dairy sectors.

Q. Are you a qualified chef, or just a great cook?

A. I'm a qualified home economist, trained in food preparation and food science, nutrition, home management, fuel studies, marketing and promotion – with a view to acting as a link between the manufacturer and the consumer.

My speciality is recipe development, recipe writing and food styling – with most of my work in the health sector.

Q. Which came first – cooking, writing, or broadcasting?

A. I've always been very domesticated. I love being in the kitchen, and even though I'm not usually working in my own – it's where I feel at home. Cooking and recipe development were natural passions of mine from a very early age – I was always experimenting and trying out new ideas, so it was just a happy coincidence to find a fantastic course to train in these skills – and combine it with a creative love of colour, texture and design – which comes to the fore with my food styling. I never tire of working with other creatives to produce beautiful images of food, that tastes great too. We shoot the food as it really is, and it's all perfectly edible.

I've always found it easy to talk about food too – whether it's in front of a live audience or broadcasting. It's the one subject where I seem to be able to retain all the facts – or quite a few, at least!

Q. What was your first piece of published work?

A. Ah, there's a story here. When I was new to freelancing, I was commissioned by a PR company to assist Keith Floyd on a presentation he was giving to cookery journalists. After he'd done his stuff, he was propping up the bar with a large glass of red. I started chatting to him and said I'd be very happy to help out again. A couple of months later he rang and left a message on my answerphone. He asked me to call his publisher. And there it began – my stroke of luck. So, having ghost-written the recipes on a few of his books, I was asked to work for Weight Watchers on their publications – and have been doing so ever since. I think I've written about 20 cook books now, but I've genuinely lost count.

Q. *How did you first get into the business of writing for the food market?*

A. I'd had three or four jobs working in the food industry, where my work as a home economist involved producing promotional literature – so I was used to slinging words together. Then when I decided to go freelance, writing became a much bigger part of the picture.

Q. *What inspires you to launch each recipe book?*

A. The inspiration comes from the commission – and what the brief is!

Q. *How do you manage to come up with so many new recipe ideas?*

A. That's a bit like asking an artist how they come up with ideas. I stare out of the window and think. I look very vacant at the time, but food ideas just churn around my head – and I make notes on possible flavour combinations. The colour, texture and design are all part of the process for me – with taste the intrinsic element. It's all in the senses. I rarely look at other books or websites for inspiration – but maybe I should!

Q. *What have been the highlights of your food writing career?*

A. It's a constant highlight to work with some great people, so it never really feels like work (though ask me again on a Friday night after a five-day shoot). It's always a thrill to see a book I've been working on come out in print – yet nothing pleases me more than when someone raves about the recipes. I once met someone who'd cooked every single recipe in *The New Dairy Cook Book* (published in 2001) – or so she said. I was so chuffed. Another time, I stayed at a fabulous bed and breakfast in Warwickshire, where the owner had masses of cookbooks. On her bookshelf was one of my Weight Watchers titles, packed full of yellow post-it notes. It turned out they were her favourite recipes – now that's a highlight.

Q. What have been the greatest challenges you've faced as a food writer?

A. Writing for Floyd was challenging. He travelled far and wide – cooking in strange and exotic places, with ingredients I had never heard of – so researching these was very time-consuming – though hugely interesting (remembering that the internet hadn't been invented then!). It was a shame there was never any budget for me to tag onto those trips.

Q. What advice would you give to budding food writers?

A. Easy – be in the right place at the right time, and speak to the right people. Seriously though, it's all about sticking with it. Perseverance is definitely the key. Don't give up – and make the most of every opportunity – you never know, you just might meet someone who can help make it happen for you.

Q. Is there anything else you'd like to share?

A. There's a lot to learn. And the only way to do it is by experience. So it's really important with food writing to research, then practise. Let other good food writers be your inspiration too.

Sue is currently working on the next Weight Watchers title, due for publication in January 2014. She has also written most of the recipes on the free downloadable app for the government's Change4Life programme, called Be Food Smart – with over 100 easy, affordable, healthy recipes. She says, "It's a great little app!"

John Negus, gardening writer

John trained as a horticulturist at Wisley Gardens and Merrist Wood Horticultural college. As a photo-journalist, he enjoys sharing his passion for gardening and other outdoor pursuits. He specialises in trees, shrubs and climbers, and lectures regularly at Grayshott Spa, gardening clubs, Women's Institutes, and many other societies. He is a member of the Surrey, Hampshire, Berkshire and Kent Federations of Judges and Lecturers, and is on the Royal Horticultural Society list of Speakers. He also lectures on board cruise liners. He broadcasts regularly on Radio Surrey and Sussex.

You will find John writing features for *Woman's Weekly* and answering queries, with a team of experts, on the *Daily Mail's* Gardening Road Shows. He answers email and snail-mail enquiries for *Amateur Gardening* and escorts groups of people around show gardens. His hobbies are gardening, photography, walking, climbing and cycling. He has written books on gardening and is an established authority in the field.

Q. Did your love of gardening open doors into the world of journalism?
A. Yes, I've always enjoyed gardening and was influenced by my granddad, who was passionate about it. But I've always loved writing too, so when we started a family and I realised we needed to up the income, I replied to an advert in Gardener's Chronicle for a technical writer. I got the job and started working for *Smallholder* magazine and *Home Gardener*. It was my first experience of commuting to London and I thought it was wonderful. Our office was next to *Country Life*, close to Covent Garden and Maiden Lane, just off the Strand. I started writing then, and I've been writing ever since.
Q. What inspired you to write each of your gardening books?
A. My first book was published in 1993 by Aura Publications. It was called Ground Cover Plants. I've also written books on garden tools, vegetables, border plants and lawns. I become passionate and evocative about each topic, and that's what inspires me to write about it.
Q. What have been the highlights of your gardening writing career?

A. I've enjoyed contributing on a regular basis to *Amateur Gardening, Homes and Gardens, Titbits* and many other magazines. The fun aspect is communicating with readers whose problems are enjoyable to solve, and helping them as much as possible. I often follow up queries by phone. It's good to make readers feel happy and know that there is a magazine that really cares about helping them.

Q. What have been the greatest challenges you've faced as a gardening writer?

A. Deadlines. I always ask for a false deadline then work to it, often when I am very tired. But it's good discipline.

Q. What advice would you give to anyone wanting to become a writer in the gardening sector?

A. You have to be dedicated to writing a feature and always do the very best you can, going through many drafts before you reach the finished article. Reading each draft is inspirational and new, and better words flood in. You have to re-read your work until every sentence, phrase and evocation fills you, and I mean you, with tingling pleasure.

Q. Is there anything else you'd like to share?

A. Writing is a great way to get to know people. It opens many doors. If you have flair, and enjoy expanding it, then commissioning editors are keen to savour it. Original thinking – that's what we gardening writers are aiming for. It's time well spent.

You can read more about John and his work at www.johnnegus.co.uk.

Helen Riches, gardening writer

Helen Riches is a gardener first, and a writer second, but her background wasn't always in gardening. She once wandered the paddy fields of China with a sketch book, designing paint tins for the Conran Group. Her background in design includes graphic design, illustration, and landscape design – inspired by ten years' developing an old neglected garden. Together, these experiences have helped Helen develop a strong eye for design and landscape gardening. Her formal education includes garden design courses at Writtle College and the College of West Anglia, as well as an honours degree in Graphic Design from Norwich School of Art. She has worked as an horticultural illustrator and says, "I find that being able to produce a garden sketch, gives clients extra confidence in ideas that they may not otherwise be able to visualise".

Q. What captured your imagination first: a love of writing or a passion for gardening?
A. I have always enjoyed writing for fun, but an interest in gardening only came when I had my own garden as an adult. Once our children were born, I stopped working as a graphic designer in order to spend more time with them. I guess gardening was an obvious creative outlet. Our garden was completely overgrown, so something had to be done!

Q. What was your first piece of published work?
A. A piece about using containers in the garden for *BBC Gardeners' World* magazine. I'd done some gardening illustrations for *BBC Gardeners' World* and I asked the art director if they would be interested in me submitting ideas as a contributor. After a couple of interviews, they said 'OK'.

Q. What have been the highlights of your gardening writing career?
A. My second published feature in 2008 won the Garden Media Guild's 'Practical Garden Journalist of the Year' Award.

Q. What have been the greatest challenges you've faced as a gardening writer?
A. My type of writing is often based on the gardening projects I develop, grow on and then explain how it's done. So my biggest challenge is keeping the plants healthy and happy until they're captured on film!

Q. What advice would you give to anyone wanting to become a writer in the gardening sector?

A. Blogging can help to build your reputation as a writer and looks like fun. I wish I had the time!

Helen's website is www.helenriches.co.uk/Writing.aspx. She also runs gardening courses.

Chapter 8

Winning pitches that resulted in a sale

There are whole books out there on how to write the perfect pitch, but I think one of the most helpful approaches, is to show you pitches that have resulted in a sale. Below are a selection of my winning pitches. Each resulted in a sale to a UK magazine, and some resulted in more than one sale.

I said earlier, that you need a 'hook', but you'll see from some of the examples below that I don't always take my own advice! A hook is not absolutely critical, but it certainly does help. It's worth remembering that articles commissioned without a reason to print imminently, may end up on the back burner for months, even years, along with your pay cheque. To give an example of what can happen when articles are accepted without being scheduled fairly quickly, one of my commissioning publications went out of print. The editor had been sitting on an article that wasn't time sensitive. The result was that the article was never published and I was never paid. That's why having your article linked to an imminent date can help.

Most of my pitches offer a degree of knowledge, or a case study that members of the editorial team are unlikely to be able to easily recreate themselves. Most explain my areas of expertise, and why I am the right person to write this particular piece.

I also add examples of where I've been published if I'm contacting an editor who I haven't worked with before.

Health pitches

The raw vegan movement: are they super-healthy, or super-nuts?
There is a growing movement of raw vegans across the world claiming that their diet can conquer any disease. Some claim to

cure cancer, whilst others only endeavour to delay the ageing process. Some say cooked food is poison to the body! It sounds too radical to be true but is there anything in it?

I will detail the benefits and myths surrounding the raw vegan diet, explaining that there are occasions when cooked food actually provides better nutrition and discuss the institutions and clinics in America which exist to cure diseased patients including those with cancer, by following a regime based primarily on raw vegan diets.

I personally tried the raw vegan diet – I'd describe the experience. I stuck to it rigidly for three months, before giving up. This is typical. Those hardliners who don't cheat are few, but there is a growing movement of enthusiasts and 'cooking' classes to fulfil the interest.

As a qualified nutritionist, I would argue that a mixed (raw and cooked) diet is best, with a little animal produce consumed for the essential nutrients it provides.

We cured his Asthma with healthy eating

My husband had asthma all through his childhood spending more time off school ill, than he spent in lessons. As he got older, his asthma continued to be a problem, and he developed an allergy to furry animals which ruled out any pets for us. Then in 2005, I took an interest in nutrition. We started eating more healthily and the change in diet cured his asthma after 47 years of anti-asthma drugs and lung-related illness. He hasn't needed any such drugs since.

We cut right down on dairy products replacing the calcium with calcium-rich vegetables and nuts instead. We cut out sugary foods, and white flour. The story covers the health benefits gained, lessons learnt, and a whole load of funny experiences along the way, which will make this a good read for anyone considering tackling their health problems with a change in diet.

Herbs of Eden

The Eden Project in Cornwall grows plants from every continent and variety, but what you don't expect to see when you visit this thriving tourist attraction, is a plot of illegal drugs! So imagine our amusement at seeing a hillside of cannabis plants next to the Tropical Biome (low drug content and licenced apparently), and then to stumble across the opiates used to produce heroin near the environmental exhibition!

For those interested in where our modern day remedies come from, both herbal and pharmaceutical, there are some enlightening plants growing in this former quarry. I'd like to take you on a tour of some of them.

Opium Poppy is an ancient source of morphine, codeine and heroin. It is farmed under licence to produce diamorphine (heroin) for medicine, where it is used in hospitals as a painkiller. Codeine in over-the-counter painkillers is also an opioid drug, producing only morphine, the precursor to heroin.

There are some interesting herbal and medical plants to draw on, including Elecampane, Fewerfew, Evening Primrose, Foxglove and Black Cohosh. I have photographs.

I would detail a lot more about the health benefits of each plant, and which part of the plant is used as a remedy. I am a qualified nutritionist and have a good background in health to write on this subject.

Ten ways to lift your spirits

'One in ten workers has taken time off because of depression' shouted the news headlines earlier this month – as if staying at home to wallow in self-pity will help the situation. I'd like to write an article on natural approaches to happiness – with a focus on lifting yourself out of depression. The first thing is to keep busy, because thinking about your problems makes them 100 times worse, so focus your mind on other things: work, hobbies, friends and exercise and keep your mind active. Some natural mood enhancers such as St John's Wort have a good reputation for alleviating depression. I'd look at food, herbs, and activities to lift your spirits, with a focus on positive thinking, and casting negative thoughts from your mind.

Milk – the big debate

There has been considerable press coverage in recent years on the health benefits of milk and its calcium-rich nutritional status.

However, milk has increasingly come under the spotlight as a food with high allergic potential. This has resulted in lactose-free milk and goats' milk appearing on our supermarket shelves.

I'd like to review the market for alternatives to cows' milk. I'd present and discuss the different types of milk available, including rice milk, oat milk, soya milk, coconut milk, and almond milk.

I'd look at their health credentials compared to dairy products, and explain how people can ensure they get sufficient calcium in their diet, regardless of which product they choose. I am a qualified nutritionist, and well placed to write this article.

Tutti Frutti

Guinea pigs love fruit and vegetables, but most children don't. I'd like to write a feature that would make fruit and vegetables seem more exciting to children. With constant references to how much guinea pigs love their vegetables, I would explain how the nutrients in fruits and vegetables keep you fit and healthy, and show how a multitude of bright colours are created by feel-good antioxidants.

This feature would look at the health benefits of children's favourite fruits, from boosting the immune system to giving you a healthy heart. It's really remarkable just how beneficial fruit and vegetables can be! The feature would conclude with interesting ways to make your vegetables taste better and how to make a banana smoothie!

Gardening pitches

Shrewsbury Flower show

We go to Shrewsbury Flower Show approximately every other year and it's a big event with some great exhibitions of HUGE vegetables, interesting varieties of tomatoes and lots of entertainment on the sidelines. Deadlines permitting, I would like to do a preview now, based on the event in previous years, with photographs, and then write a review, by attending the event in August, and reporting back on it for a later issue in September/October. Complete with lots of photographs of the fruit and vegetable exhibits.

The medicinal benefits of your herb plot

I wondered if you'd like something on garden herbs and their medicinal properties? I have pics of some of these:

- Sage leaf prepared as an herbal tea can help to settle indigestion, boost appetite, and reduce the effect of hot flushes.
- Nettle tea is great for the liver.
- Mint helps to settle an irritable bowel and can be used as a dressing, to spice up a salad, or served as an herbal tea.
- Rosemary tea is a pick-me-up for a modest burst of energy.
- Arnica is used in commercial creams for bringing out and reducing bruising. The herb is harmful if swallowed, but rubbing the leaves onto a bruise may produce the same benefit as a commercial preparation.
- The leaves of the Globe Artichoke are well known in France as a bitter digestive remedy after heavy meals and there is evidence that it increases bile flow, improves digestion, and even lowers cholesterol.
- Fennel is a great addition to any salad and it contains phytonutrients which keep hormones in check and protect

against some cancers. The seeds can relax the intestines and reduce bloating.

Upcycling: transforming rubbish into something useful!

Are you interested in a feature on upcycling in the garden? It's about reusing items which might otherwise go to landfill, to fulfil a purpose in your garden? And it has the potential to save readers some money too – a good idea in these hard-hitting times? From water butts to pots and planters, upcycling is the latest fad in environmental activism, and many gardeners have been doing it for years!

Examples include:

- turning barrels into water butts
- a planter into a birdbath
- coleslaw cartons transformed into slug pubs
- using paving slabs to make a duck island
- old timber decking to make a duck house
- timber decking used to create steps for a path over a waterfall
- an unwanted tub transformed into a guinea pig shelter
- and plastic bottles over your young plants.

I'd speak to a variety of gardeners to get their innovative uses for upcycling old items in their garden, and lots of photographs to accompany the article.

Attingham Park

I have just returned from Shropshire where we visited Attingham Park and its glorious kitchen garden. The garden is being renovated, and they are more than half way through the project having recreated the Victorian vegetable garden with a wide range of produce. They have melons in their greenhouses, held up in little pouches that look like ladies' bras! They have a thriving bee population in one of only two grade II listed beehives in Britain. The volunteer beekeeper says they send samples of the honey off to DEFRA to find out from which plant the pollen originates. On one occasion, years ago, the scientists were left scratching their heads and delays occurred as they tried to figure out what the bees had been feeding on. Eventually, the answer came back: Coca Cola.

The wonderful scent of basil hits you as you enter one of the greenhouses. The water well was excavated last summer and used to be the main source of water for the garden. It is slowly filling up. They also plan to restore the dipping pond which used to be filled from the well and provided slightly warmer water for the garden.

A quarter of the walled garden has been taken over by a labyrinth. The gardeners spend most of their mornings picking, sorting, and weighing fresh salads and vegetables for the tea room and shop. Bare ground where harvesting has been completed, is covered by red clover and alfalfa just to keep the weeds down and to be worked back into the soil in the spring.

The main garden leads into a second smaller kitchen garden, where the greenhouses are, along with lots of ripe and tasty fruit, and then into an orchard with chickens that just love to wallow in the mud. There is an exhibition of a Victorian gardener's house and how he would have lived, as well as the original record book of the planting scheme 100-odd years ago.

The house is worth a visit whilst you're there. A Georgian lady (tour guide) will tell you about the son who inherited the estate and then through a series of excessive expenditures, and political rivalries, went into bankruptcy after which the whole estate and its contents were auctioned to repay his debts.

Erddig's Fruit Garden

We recently visited Erdigg House in Wales, a big old mansion house with a large garden that grows fruit along all the walls and in the huge orchards. They had trouble with looters back in the early 20th century when they put up signs (for anyone who could read) to say they would be reprimanded for trespassing and nicking the fruit.

The fruit lives on today, with hundreds of bushes of every variety of apple, plum, and pear as well as fig bushes, grape vines, and berries. I wonder if you would be interested in a piece about this fruit garden, the family that lived there, their troubles with looters, and the house and grounds as a visitor attraction today. I'd catch up with the head gardener and ask him about the highlights and challenges of working on the estate. They also have bees. Pictures attached.

Food

Growing onions for health

Onions are an incredibly healthy food. Natural antifungals and with mild antibiotic properties, they have also been shown to provide a degree of protection against arthritis, cardiovascular disease, and inflammatory conditions. Onions are loaded with antioxidants, and taken fresh from your garden, they maintain their maximum nutritional content better than supermarket produce which has been stored and transported. The health claims are supported by recent scientific studies and I would provide a nutritional breakdown for onions, looking at the benefits of these nutrients all working in combination. I would suggest finishing with a recipe or two for onion bhajis and cheese and onion quiche. I can provide pictures of onions and the recipes cooked and ready to eat.

Summer salads

As the hot weather kicks in, Nutritionist Susie Kearley looks at some healthy summer salads which you can create, mostly from home-grown produce.

Salads can be very filling if you think big and add beans or pasta to the mix. Try adding fruits and nuts to make them varied and interesting. Salads are one of the most nutritionally dense dishes available because they are mostly raw, meaning none of the nutrients are lost during cooking and processing. I'd include recipes for bean salad, fruity salad, and home-made coleslaw. Pictures supplied.

Growing garlic for health

Garlic is a potent health provider that has been shown to improve the balance of good bacteria in the gut. Garlic can slow or reverse the early effects of Alzheimer's disease, reduce cholesterol, fight infections, and boost immunity. I would quote scientific studies to support these claims, and would break down the nutritional content of Garlic, showing how the nutrients working together have benefits that outweigh individual nutrients alone. I would suggest completing the article with a recipe for a favourite garlic-based recipe or two – pesto with garlic bread, and garlic-stuffed olives. I can provide pictures of garlics and of the recipes cooked and ready to eat. I am a qualified nutritionist and freelance writer.

Make your own healthy chocolate snacks for Valentine's Day

Healthy chocolate balls? Yes, these sugar-free delights are sweetened with dates and raisins. They contain cholesterol-lowering oats, antioxidant-rich cocoa powder, healthy nuts, and they're quick to make, and delicious!

For those people wanting to enjoy chocolate in a healthy way on Valentine's Day, this is a winner! I propose to write a feature where I would detail the health benefits of these surprisingly filling chocolate snacks, and explain how chocolate balls can provide an alternative to fattening novelty chocolates, without breaking the healthy eating plan!

Healthy Christmas treats

As Christmas nears, your healthy eating is destined to go out the window. But when you're eating at home, or entertaining friends, you can provide healthy options and might be surprised just how well they go down!

I've created my own recipe for healthy mince pies – without sugar or sweeteners, they are sweetened only by the natural fruit sugars that the pies contain. Made with wholemeal flour (or my preference is rye flour) they are a greater source of nutrients than traditional mince pies, providing manganese and fibre to support your joints and your bowel health respectively.

They are also rich in natural antioxidants from the fruit and this makes them good for your heart. I'd use olive oil in the pastry, which is a healthy fat. It's all about choosing healthy ingredients for this tasty dessert, finished with a dollop of natural probiotic yogurt, or just eaten cold – delicious!

I'd also look at other healthy eating options for the Christmas period to include: vegetable dips, lots of salad, and a home-made quiche which always goes down well in a Christmas buffet.

Exercise

Try writing a good pitch of your own. Think of a topic you are strong on, add a current 'hook', an interviewee, detail your qualifications and experience, and create a winning pitch to a magazine of your choice.

Chapter 9

Conducting interviews

I like writing interview pieces. Generally, I find them one of the easiest and most rewarding assignments. They get me out meeting new people, which is nice because freelance writing can be a lonely profession at times. However, some people find conducting interviews quite difficult, so here are some pointers to help you get the most from your interview opportunities.

Preparing questions

Not sure where to start, or what to ask? Prepare a list of questions in advance – this is good practice. But don't be too much of a stickler for the questions you've prepared – they should be a prompt, a reminder, something to move the interview along – not a burden to be imposed upon your interviewee at any cost. Sometimes interviewers become so focused on the questions that they forget to listen properly to the answers!

Your questions need to be open ended, and almost impossible to answer with a yes or no. Sit down beforehand and think about what you want to know, and what the magazine's readers would be interested in. Write down key questions and don't be afraid to ask your interviewee to elaborate on their answers.

If you want to find out how someone survived cancer by switching to a raw vegan lifestyle, ask them to reveal the details of their daily regime if that's what would interest the readers. Dig in, ask questions and listen hard, taking extensive notes, or with the aid of a Dictaphone.

You often don't need many questions because once they start talking it all comes out, but it's helpful to have 10-20 questions prepared in advance. This provides a checklist to ensure you've got all you need before you let them go, and it gives you some questions to get them talking again if they do dry up.

Interesting but unexpected answers can take the interview in a different direction, and elicit additional instinctive questions on different topics altogether. I've done interviews where my original list of questions got discarded half way through!

If the conversation moves off in a different direction it can make your article more interesting – revealing things you hadn't thought of, and angles you hadn't considered. Don't be afraid to follow a different route if that's how the interview goes, as long as it doesn't veer off topic altogether, to subjects that are not within the broad scope of your brief.

Icebreakers

If you are struggling to get started with an interviewee because they seem cold and unresponsive, it can be useful to some have icebreakers in mind. Asking people to tell you about their pets tends to warm people up, especially if they are nervous. This approach will make them feel more comfortable – warming them up for when you ask the more difficult questions later.

Many years ago, I had a job interview for a marketing position within a small consulting firm. I was dead nervous. The interviewer called me in, sat me down, and said, "So you've got guinea pigs?" He smiled, and added, "We used to have guinea pigs too!" It broke the ice in an instant and I told him their names, and elaborated a little – they were from a rescue centre. Before I knew it, we were talking about the garden pond! Whether to use this approach depends very much on your interviewee, how pushed for time they are, and whether they need an icebreaker.

Now I'll be honest – I've never had to use an icebreaker in journalism yet. I just storm straight in and it seems to work fine. But maybe I've been lucky. In many cases, I am interviewing a person who is passionate about their topic, so it's easy to get them to talk. People love talking about their favourite hobbies and things they are enthusiastic about.

Double checking in health interviews

You might find in the field of health, practitioners are often keen to double check what you have written about them or quoted, because if you get it wrong, it could affect their reputation, or they could be accused of offering bad health advice, which might come back to haunt them. So I'd particularly recommend getting health practitioners to check over your manuscript when you quote them as a source.

What's the best way to conduct an interview?

I conduct my interviews in a variety of ways. Face-to-face is invariably the best approach, but rarely practical for reasons of distance, travel, and time. Many of my interviews are, therefore, conducted by telephone, but I'm increasingly leaning towards emails, where people have time to think through their answers and complete the questions at their own pace. The reason I'm starting to do more this way, is because it's the way a lot of people prefer to work. And to be honest, it makes life easier for me too, because I get the first draft delivered to my computer, all typed up. The down side is that some interviewees can't spell, can't punctuate, and the word structuring might be terrible. Sometimes it needs to be completely re-hashed and sent back for approval. This can mean it's easier to transcribe notes from an interview – because having spoken to them and clarified some points, my notes make more sense!

However, emailed responses are rarely that bad and I still usually find it easiest to have the interviewee's written answers there in front of me. Let's look at the options – I'd suggest you try each of them yourself to find out what works best for you.

Face-to-face interviews

The best interviews are usually done face-to-face and if you're going to speak to your local health practitioner for an interview piece, then this method is probably convenient too.

A face-to-face interview helps you both relax and can bring out the best in your interviewee. It is also possible to get much more from the conversation, when you are there in the room with them. Descriptions of their body language, reactions, interruptions and even your surroundings can all add to the vibrancy of your article, as it helps readers to imagine the interview taking place, and relate to the conversation and the atmosphere.

You can describe the ambience of the health clinic, the style of the treatment room and what the practitioner looked like. You might get a free treatment, to enable you to describe how the therapy made you feel. All this adds to an interview piece, enabling the reader to build a picture in their mind.

Face-to-face interviews offer scope to insert humour too. You can write about the funny things that happen when you're interviewing people – the things you laugh about together, and the things they probably didn't intend to say, but let you print anyway. It enables you to reflect their personality more accurately than other methods of interview and incorporates the bigger picture, even down to the details of arriving for the interview stressed or soaked by rain.

Describing the environment can really bring an interview piece to life.

Last year, I went to see dog trainer Jackie Prescott, who appeared on Britain's Got Talent with her dancing dog Tippy Toes, reaching the semi-finals in 2009. We sat on the dog-chewed sofa (literally), with foam pouring out the sides, and were surrounded by four enthusiastic dogs, and ten bunnies. As you can imagine the completed interview piece contained a lot more than Jackie's quotes. The whole environment came to life.

You can use a Dictaphone or a notepad. If you don't know shorthand, you might struggle to get enough words down on a notepad, but I've developed my own version of shorthand which helps.

However, you may prefer the freedom that a Dictaphone

gives you – it enables you to focus completely on the interviewee and the environment, rather than messing around with a notepad and pen, trying to keep up with the pace of chat. The downside of using a Dictaphone is all the transcription required when you get home. It can take ages and personally, I much prefer a notepad and pen, which enables me to type up my notes quite quickly when I get home. Some writers who prefer to use a Dictaphone pay other people to transcribe their recordings because they don't have time for all the transcription afterwards.

If your face-to-face interviewee starts rambling away from the topic in hand, and the diversion is tiresome, bring them back gently. I don't find rambling too much of a problem in the health, food, and gardening markets – generally interviewees in these areas tend to stick to the point. But I have had very rambling interviews in other areas of my work, and I've found that one way to reduce the rambling is to do the interview by telephone.

Telephone interviews

When you are not able to meet your interviewee face-to-face, the telephone does provide an opportunity to get some of that unspoken feedback that brings a story to life – laughter, uncomfortable pauses, comments they say to you in person, but wouldn't necessarily write down because they don't think it's relevant or important.

You get an instantaneous response to questions, which, depending on your topic, could make for a better interview than responses that they've had time to ponder over.

That said, I have found, that during telephone interviews, they will tell you one thing, and then during the proofreading stage, they'll change their story and ask for those little things to change or come out. One recent example was when I was interviewing a Druid who told me over the phone that he didn't believe in any of the pagan gods. At the proofreading stage, he wanted that comment changed to say that he did. I think he felt the comment was too controversial and to be a practising Druid who doesn't believe in the pagan gods is not the 'done thing'.

You don't have to show your interviewees a proof, but I prefer to get approval from all my interviewees, even if it is at the expense of a few lighthearted remarks. I want them to be happy with what I've written about them, and if that means we lose a little something in the editing process, to be honest, it rarely matters... and sometimes they can be persuaded to leave it in anyway!

If you do get an interviewee who is very long-winded over the telephone, you need to gently steer them back to the key points in hand and politely keep them on track. I had one telephone interview recently with a chap who had so much to say that I could have written a small book based on his interview. Suffice to say, many of his ramblings couldn't be included in the article, and what was included, was severely cut. For a while, I let him ramble, and after two very long calls, I wrote the article and sent it back for his approval.

He responded with another four long telephone calls, each time wanting to include dozens of other points for which we simply didn't have the space. I persistently had to stress that point, but we did pull a few things out and added new things in, to ensure that the article communicated everything that he felt was important. It was a long and drawn out process for an article that was only ever intended to be submitted on spec! That's certainly something I'd never plan to do, but fortunately, the article was accepted. Now, if I have the inclination for further dealings with this enthusiastic gentleman, I have enough material for at least another two or three articles!

You might want to rein your interviewees in a little more than I did for that piece – it ultimately depends on how useful the additional information is likely to be, and how firm you're prepared to be with someone who's running away with enthusiasm for his subject!

One of the key benefits of interviewing people either face-to-face, or by telephone, is that you don't have to stick to the questions that you started with. You can wander off on tangents to all sorts of areas that you didn't even know you wanted to know about. If these diversions are not useful for the article in hand, they sometimes provide material for another project. However, they can also make the interview much more interesting.

Take the example of Jackie Prescott again. When I first contacted her, I didn't know that she been on Britain's Got Talent. I just knew she had a dancing dog and was opening a 'charm school' for dogs locally. Only by interviewing her face-to-face, did I find out that she'd been in one of the biggest shows on television! And then of course I started asking her about that experience, which wasn't on my list of original questions at all!

Email interviews

The third approach to interviewing, is to send the questions to your interviewees and let them reply by email in their own time. This is the easiest approach in many ways as they essentially prepare the first draft of your article for you. You don't necessarily get their initial response, but you do get a considered response. The downside is that the considered response is often very long and needs considerable work in editing.

I've also had the situation where someone agreed to answer a few questions by email because he didn't want to be interviewed by phone or in person. He then provided one or two word answers to all my open ended questions. They were designed to be impossible to answer in one word – yet somehow he managed it!

You give away the power when you give away your questions, and getting the answers you want in the length you require is rare. However, fortunately, most people over-write and cutting is much easier than fudging an interview piece that consists of one-word answers. So if you don't mind some heavy cutting, and this approach suits you both, it can work very well. I use it quite a lot. That said, some interviewees deliver the perfect piece by email. I interviewed the herbalist and prolific author, Anne McIntyre, about the health benefits of different herbs and what they are used for. Her answers were exactly the right length and depth for my piece. It may of course help that she is a writer herself so she knew what I was looking for.

I do have myself to blame for sometimes getting unduly long responses from enthusiastic interviewees. I rarely tell them how long a piece should be because I don't want to constrain them, and I'm very happy to cut down their words afterwards if necessary. After all, making the words fit into the article is my job, not theirs. Sometimes it doesn't matter how long the interviews are, because the brief is pretty flexible anyway. I'd rather have the full story and trim it afterwards than have a story that's not as interesting as it might have been.

With email interviews, you may have to go back to your source to clarify one or two points, as you don't have the opportunity to get clarification in the moment. That opportunity for immediate clarity is another key benefit of interviewing by telephone or in person. But don't rule out email. It can be a great way to pull everyone's answers together when you're busy.

Keep hold of your evidence

After you have completed your interview and written up your copy, it is advisable to hang onto the recording, notes, emails and other evidence associated with the article until you know that no one's going to come back and challenge you on it. Once the article is published and you know your sources are happy with what has been written you can probably relax, but depending on the content, it might be advisable to hang onto your evidence for a bit longer.

Be organised and file away all your email communications,

digital recordings, or written notes, as well as your typed transcript of the conversation. It's something to fall back on if the source, or anyone else, objects to what has been written.

Interviews do hold potential for objections more than some other articles because you are quoting people directly – and people are prone to changing their story! That's why I prefer to run my completed copy past my interviewee, prior to submitting it to the editor. After all, if they don't like what I say about them, or I quote them saying something that they later disagree about, there is the potential for conflict, and even for legal action.

Interviewees often change their mind about what they want to appear in the article, between talking to you and seeing the proposed final copy of the interview transcript written up for a magazine.

Even when they have approved what you submit, hang on to their emails saying it's fine. That way, if they come back later and say they didn't agree to it, you have their email, showing that they did.

I've never actually had anybody come back and complain about what I've written about them, possibly because I have been very careful in this respect. When someone is kind enough to cooperate with me and help me with my writing, then I give them due respect, and usually let them see the final copy before I send it in. This does result in a few tweaks, but nothing major – and rarely does this have any big impact on the final article. It also means that this person has confidence in me in the future, and will cooperate with future articles where I need an interviewee. That's a valuable resource to have on hand.

Exercise

Think about times when you have been in an interview situation, perhaps for a job or a place at college. Did the interviewer use any special techniques to put you at ease?

Now write down some people that you would like to

interview for your writing, and jot down some open ended questions that you'd like to ask them. Practise on a friend or relative if you're not very confident. Interviewing really is quite easy when you get used to it.

Chapter 10

Food and garden photography

Both food and gardening magazines often demand high-quality pictures as an essential part of the package when they commission an article. This is particularly important for recipes, as it goes without saying that the dish has to look tasty, and you have to have a great picture every time.

So do you have the skills and the equipment to rise to this challenge? Perhaps surprisingly, you don't need copious amounts of either, but a basic appreciation of what they're looking for and what works, definitely helps.

Artistically, you'll notice that many of the pictures in food magazines are of beautifully laid out table settings and exquisitely prepared food. They usually have a sharp focus on the foreground – the dish – and soft focus on the background. The photographer has paid great attention to the layout, sometimes even employing a food stylist to set the table scene while he or she focuses on the lighting and shooting angles. These are all things that you need to pay attention to if you want to focus your writing interests on the food and cookery market.

For some magazines you can get away with a simple snapshot looking down at a dish from above. This requires very little in the way of scene setting and table preparation. But you still need to make sure it's sharp and you have good lighting.

This simple approach is exactly how I began writing for the food markets with a small compact digital camera, and a plate of home-made food.

The difference between elaborate table settings and really quite simple shots, may be significant in the different types of magazine that you find yourself able to work for. My early cookery photos were fine for many gardening magazines, women's magazines and smallholding publications, but they were unlikely to be accepted by glossy specialist recipe magazines, where the recipe is the main feature, and their readers are used to perfect dinner settings and soft focus tableware.

Last year I upgraded my camera, purchasing an entry level DSLR, and then went on a course to learn how to use it.

We began learning about apertures and shutter speeds. A wide aperture is what enables you to focus on the food and achieve that attractive soft background. Some more expensive compact cameras do enable you to take pictures with a wide aperture, but many only have small lenses which by their nature, limit you to a narrow aperture – essentially meaning that every-thing is in sharp focus most of the time. A budget compact camera provides little scope to create that selective soft focus that is popular in recipe magazines, so if you want to create that effect, you may need to spend a bit more.

Getting the perfect shot

If you are targeting the glossy recipe magazines then the layout of your food can't be stressed enough. Tidy up before you cook and prepare your table setting and lighting, so that once the food is cooked, you're ready to shoot.

A food photographer I once knew, always said you need to be prepared to let the food get cold while you get the perfect shot. You may need to set up artificial lighting with three or four lamps, or to take time with the table arrangements.

Other people working in the industry, seem to be able to get their lighting set up in advance, then quickly shoot and eat. You can experiment to find out what works for you.

For my gardening photography I take hundreds of photographs, including gardener action shots, and close ups of flowers, insects and vegetables. You may also find you have to pose for shots or buy vegetables from the supermarket when the produce you're writing about has failed to grow on your own plot, or is out of season. I recently had to set up a scene for a photo shoot that looked like I'd just grown a load of vegetables in March. Many of the vegetables that made it into the final photo shoot, had just been imported to our local supermarket from Spain!

One editor, after clarifying his instructions on how a gardening article should take shape, added: "Also a selection of good pics. One of you with a spade digging in the garden, or outdoors holding a selection of veg in your arms/a trug/a veg box and looking into the camera. That would be brilliant too. Produce can be shop-bought of course, but mustn't look like it!"

So as a freelance writer in this market, you need to be a jack of all trades – artist, food stylist, photographer, interviewer, horticulturalist, garden pest controller, health practitioner (or know someone who is), fitness guru and cook!

Camera settings

Details like selecting the right light setting on your camera to cope with different lighting conditions, can make quite a big difference to your finished picture. When you're taking pictures of the garden in the sun, you'll need a different setting to when you're taking shots of a table setting under artificial light. It's a good idea to make sure you're aware of how to find these different settings on your DSLR camera. There's usually a fluorescent light setting, a sunlight and a shady setting – and there are different ISO settings, which allow different amounts of light into the lens.

If you have a budget compact, don't worry as it's probably all automatic (or only has one setting), but if you have a DSLR then there are all sorts of little enhancements that you should become familiar with, to improve your photography.

I'd recommend getting yourself onto a photography course as exploring the different features of your camera with an expert tutor can really help. Even if you get there and find that you know most of it, you're bound to pick up a few useful tips along the way and maybe you could sell an article about the course! If you're already trading as a freelance writer, then any training that you purchase after you have started trading is tax deductible in the UK.

Digital enhancement

Digital enhancement is another great tool in the photographer's armoury. It enables you to turn a picture that's disappointingly dark, into a bright image, fit for purpose. However, digital enhancement has its limitations, so don't rely on it too much. It's much better to work on getting that perfect shot in situ, and to keep digital enhancements to a minimum.

I find Photoshop Elements is a cheap and intuitive package, but you can also download Gimp for free, which has some great features. Playing with the levels, contrast and colour slides can help you perfect your work. The clone tool can help to remove unwanted items in the picture, but done badly, cloning is really obvious, so keep the cloning to a minimum unless you're really skilled at it.

What does 300 dpi mean?

You'll quickly come across the term 300 dpi when you start talking about photographs to editors. 300 dpi means 300 dots per inch. In plain English, this means they want a high resolution image. Exactly how high resolution? Well that depends how big they want to print your image – information you can never know, so it's always advisable to set your digital camera on the highest resolution possible and leave it there. On a decent camera, that should provide a photograph large enough for a full page spread, and possibly for a double page spread.

If you've provided the highest resolution photographs that your equipment allows, then this is helpful, giving the publisher maximum flexibility on the layout without having to worry about poor-quality, pixelated images.

They may want to print your picture as a double page spread, or crop your photo and focus on a small part of the image, so they'll need a high resolution file to achieve a good result. That's why leaving your camera set on its highest resolution makes sense.

As a minimum, a 1mb file is usually acceptable. As long as your pictures are at least 1mb, before digital enhancement, they should be fine for most purposes (digital enhancement increases the size of the file but not the resolution).

The other problem I sometimes find is when you get an interviewee who does a wonderful interview, but then provides a photograph of themselves that is 30kb. This can be a problem if they live miles away so you can't go and take one easily. You may have to go back to your interviewee and push them for a larger file to prevent the image coming out highly pixelated in print, or being rejected altogether. I've only had one person who was unable to provide a bigger shot, and due to the distance and her complete inability to get one taken at her end, we're having to work with what we've got. I suspect the editor might ditch the head shot altogether when that particular piece comes out. You might get away with this on a small press magazine, but don't think for a minute, you can get away with shoddy photos for a high circulation, glossy publication. In fact, if they're among the market leaders, they might require a professional photo shoot and supply the photographer.

Photography Copyright

Never download photographs off the internet and submit them to illustrate an article unless you have the express permission from the owner of the copyright to do so. The fact that an image is on the internet, does not mean it is free to use by anyone. The idea that anything posted online is free to use, or 'in the public domain' is nonsense. Photography and words posted online are still protected by copyright laws. You can end up with huge bills for breach of copyright if you're not careful.

'Public domain' is a term used to describe material for which the copyright has expired, either because the author has been dead for 70 years, or because copyright doesn't apply – as is the case with some official government documents.

The UK Government Intellectual Property Office says: 'Protection for an original written, theatrical, musical or artistic work lasts for the life of the creator plus 70 years from the end of the year in which he/she died.'

If you think receiving a huge bill for copyright infringement is unlikely, let me tell you a true story about an incident that occurred during my former marketing career in 2009. I received a letter from Getty Images (who supply the BBC and other significant names with their photographs), demanding payment for unauthorised use of one of their photographs. They directed me to a website where this alleged breach had occurred. It was a website branded with my organisation, but not one that, until this moment, I knew existed. When I queried it with my boss, he said he thought the site had been closed down years ago!

Anyway, it transpired that a previous member of staff had taken the photograph off the internet to illustrate the page with no concern for the owner of the photograph or for the breach of copyright. No one questioned it, so the image stayed up there for years.

That legal demand cost our department around £1000. Don't underestimate how much breach of copyright can cost you – and your editor, who trusts you to come up with either photography that you own, or authorised shots, complete with permission to use them and suitable credits to the copyright holder.

Prosecution for copyright theft does happen. Use your own photographs where possible. Apart from copyright issues, photos downloaded from the internet are rarely high resolution enough for print publication, so even if you do have permission, you usually need to go chasing higher resolution copies from the copyright owner.

The other thing of which you should be aware, is the consequence if your publisher fails to credit the photographer when using third party photos with permission. Stress the credits to them, and put it in the image title to remind the designer. Publishers do sometimes forget to credit the photographs when they print them, and then you have a potential copyright issue to deal with, and lots of apologising to do. Failure to comply with the conditions of use (proper crediting) could result in a hefty bill. For example, the BBC sometimes lets you use photographs of TV programmes if you credit them correctly. If the magazine subsequently uses them but fails to credit them correctly, it can cost a small fortune – all completely unnecessarily.

Photography clubs

Photography clubs will stretch your skills, help you see what works and what doesn't and pit your work against others in the club which helps you to see how your photography can be improved. It's worth joining a photography club if you're serious about doing photography as part of your writing work, because it's bound to help raise your standards, and to help you gain hints and tips on composition, digital enhancement, and what makes a cracking photograph.

Exercise

Try setting up a table place, with a tempting dish as a centrepiece that would look great in a foodie magazine. Then experiment with lighting and camera angles to get a variety of different shots that might be suitable for publication. Next, take your camera outside and take photographs of a garden – whether it's your own garden or a stately home, it doesn't matter. Again, experiment with different angles and get a collection of macro shots, to help you get the best results and to learn from practising.

Chapter 11

Turning rejections into an acceptance

When I started writing for the food, health and gardening markets it was a rocky road, littered with disappointment and rejection. But fortunately, with perseverance and determination, I've since sold thousands of articles to publishers across the globe. One thing I have learnt to do however, is master the art of turning rejections into opportunities, some of which have resulted in sales. Here are some of the lessons I've learnt.

Lesson 1: Give the editor what he or she wants

Take 3! The sound of eggs sizzling in the frying pan filled the air and James, the editor of *Good Motoring* magazine, asked: "What do you think of my breakfast this morning, Susie?"

He poked a microphone at my face and I garbled something incoherent about fry ups not being very nutritious. Porridge would be better.

We were recording a podcast for the Good Motoring website, and the 'cooking breakfast' sounds were pre-recorded.

I was nervous and didn't like being unprepared. I wanted to write my answers down and read them back with confidence, but James whipped my notepad away saying he didn't want it to sound staged. "No danger of that," I thought.

The interview was the outcome of a rejection letter. James had rejected my proposal to write about the hair-raising experience of being a learner motorcyclist on British roads, but said he was interested in other road safety ideas. So instead, I secured a commission to write about good nutrition to help drivers concentrate on the road – this podcast was part of the package.

"I don't normally eat a full English breakfast," said James, "but I thought it would give us more to talk about!" And so began the start of a beautiful working relationship – he has since bought my articles on speed cameras and motorcycle driving tests too.

What did I learn from this experience? To listen and learn from the feedback received. Look for opportunities that rejection letters reveal and then give the editor what he wants.

Lesson 2: Don't write an essay!

One of my earliest customers was *Paranormal* magazine. The editor, Brian, didn't offer firm commissions, but would tell me if he liked an idea. Then I'd submit a full article on spec for his consideration.

He was interested in an idea I'd pitched entitled 'The Psychology of Fear' so I trawled through my psychology degree books, writing up all things fear-related including conditions like panic attacks and their treatment. It was well researched but a bit academic, so I made an attempt to lighten it up and submitted it.

Brian rejected the piece saying it was 'too clinical'. More suited to a psychology journal than a magazine about hauntings. I understood the problem and managed to find another buyer for some of the work: *Leader* magazine is an academic title published by the Association of Schools and Colleges. I used some of the 'fear' material in a feature on stress and it worked well because the body's reactions to stress are very similar to fear.

Leader paid three times as much as *Paranormal*, and the sale resulted in commissions for a further two articles on the topics of nutrition and social media.

What I learnt: If you write something on spec which is rejected, think laterally about alternative markets for the piece, and consider whether parts of the article could be used to cover a different topic altogether. Rejected work can still form the basis of a good article for a different market, and that can lead to a profitable long-term relationship.

Lesson 3: Get the presentation right

I came across a very sad story about a gentleman called Jim, who suddenly lost his sight, but then turned his life around and triumphed over adversity in a really inspirational way. In the months following the onset of his blindness, Jim was transformed from a taxi-driver who thought his life was over, to an inspirational figurehead for the blind community. He had an active lifestyle doing diverse sporting activities, and mastering incredible achievements against the odds. Jackie, the editor of *Woman Alive*, told me she would be interested in seeing his story written speculatively.

So I fixed an interview with Jim and his wife Ellen, sat down and asked them about their experiences. They both chipped in and were bouncing stories off one another, giving slightly different perspectives. I submitted the interview piece just like that, with both Jim and Ellen chipping in, but Jackie said she needed their stories told separately from two different perspectives – it's a woman's magazine, and Ellen's story should be longer.

So I went back to the drawing board and produced two separate interviews. I also livened it up, and went to check with Jim and Ellen that I hadn't over-sensationalised it. No, they said it was fine – the whole experience really was dramatic and traumatic so I hadn't overdone it!

The two interviews worked well and Jackie was delighted with the result. She has since commissioned many more articles including the healing power of nutrition and healthy Christmas treats!

What I learnt: Make sure you have an appreciation of what's expected, and if you get it wrong the first time, correct it. Take time to make sure it's good. You may not get a third opportunity.

Chapter 12

Freelancing for PR firms

Some magazines, particularly in the health sector, don't pay for material but are quite happy to take articles written by journalists working on behalf of public relations companies. This may not be your first choice of work, and the product you are required to promote may not be your preferred treatment for a health complaint, but it's an option to consider. In these circumstances, it is possible to promote the product, alongside your best dietary and therapeutic recommendations, whilst keeping everyone happy and securing payment from a PR firm. This approach enables you to work for magazines that don't pay, while still making money out of it.

I don't work for PR firms directly, although I have had non-paying magazines (who at the time of pitching I thought might pay) tell me that they'd like to take the article (for free) if I can get sponsorship from a PR company. Luckily for me, I've always been too busy with freelance work to need to chase PR companies for business, but it is something to consider if things get quiet.

On a similar note, I have also been asked by commissioning editors who do pay their freelance writers, to promote certain products within my wider health article. This is because the editor has a connection with the company and wants to offer them some coverage, for whatever reason – perhaps they are a good advertiser.

One recent example was an article about detoxification. I was asked to mention the current trend in 'fasting' diets, where you cut down to 500 calories 2 days a week. The editor wanted me to include a very expensive syrup product as an alternative to eating 500 calories of solid food on these days. I felt it would be much better for readers to eat 500 calories of fruit and vegetables, but to meet the editor's requirements, I had to include the syrup as an option too. It went in a sidebar, as an alternative approach to getting your 500 calories a day on 'fast' days.

The way to approach articles where you are asked to promote a product that perhaps you don't entirely agree with, is to offer a wider array of suggestions for managing your health complaint, whilst giving the product a place among them.

Taking joint pain as an example, you might include the company's product, but might also include dietary measures, relaxing baths, and gentle exercise, so that it is broadly an independent article, giving genuinely helpful suggestions based on your reading, qualifications, and experience, whilst at the same time, mentioning the company's product, as per your brief.

It is important if you are being paid to promote products, to be up front with your editor about any PR connections/bias in your article. Magazines who don't pay for articles generally expect a degree of bias – writers have to earn their money some how. If the magazine won't pay, then this approach is inevitable.

This approach can lead to you working more as a freelance public relations executive, than a journalist, but it still provides opportunities to use your creative talents, write and get paid for it. There is no shame in that as long as you're honest with editors about it.

Magazines that don't pay for submissions are also an easy target because other freelancers aren't knocking on their door so much. This means there's a greater likelihood of your idea being accepted. The magazines who operate like this are typically small press magazines, with very little money behind them, and they are often advertising led. They appeal to niche markets and rely heavily on advertising.

In the alternative health markets, there are so many niche areas – crystal healing, shamanic healing, Native American traditions, nutritional therapy, acupuncture, Chinese herbal medicine, angelic healing therapies, reflexology, reiki… the list goes on and on, with new alternative health practices emerging every day.

Numerous small press magazines focus on their own unique brand of health and healing. Some of them rely on enthusiasts to write for free, because they are not in a position to pay. They include yoga magazines, charity magazines, free giveaway magazines at health stores, and some very specialist spiritual publications. Many are interested in receiving articles based on new products and PR material.

There is no reason why you shouldn't write public relations articles for gardening magazines too – there are many manufac-turers and suppliers of garden equipment that would no doubt, be pleased to have a double page spread on how their products can solve gardeners' problems. I have come across fewer publica-tions that don't pay journalists in this sector however – so they may be less willing to accept material with a PR bias. The same goes for food magazines.

The danger of working as a journalist and in public relations is that you may be asked by your PR company to write an article that you can't place with a publication – and your pay depends on it being published. Don't write it. I usually only write an article that an editor has, at a minimum, expressed a genuine interest in publishing. More often, I have a firm commission. Working on a piece for a PR company, without any expression of interest from a publisher could turn out to be a complete waste of time.

Once you have ascertained interest from an editor, write the article with that publication in mind, taking into account their house style. Unless it's a firm commission, there are no guarantees it will be accepted, but it does mean the editor will look favourably upon your completed contribution, and if all goes well, your piece will be printed and you'll get paid by the PR firm.

The other reason that some specialists write for magazines that don't pay, is if they are building up their reputation and promoting their business. If you recall, Jackie Lynch, the nutritionist and health writer, employed a PR expert to get her space in some big name publications so that she could develop her published profile, promote her nutrition business and make a name for herself.

This opened up opportunities to write for some high profile glossy publications as their qualified 'expert', usually quoted within someone else's article. It can help to raise your profile and hone your writing skills, but you are unlikely to earn much from the experience, and as Jackie found out, it can be quite expensive. However, if you gain a good reputation and new skills from the experience, it may lead to publications commissioning you as an expert freelance writer in your own right. That's what's happened to Jackie, who having established herself as an expert published in some big name magazines, has started to earn from writing her own articles too.

Exercise

Write down which product ranges would fit nicely into your knowledge pool and which publications might be interested in stories of this nature. Jot down a few story ideas, and when you're ready to approach the PR office for your favourite brand range, you'll have some ideas already brewing and can build upon them if the response is positive. You need to sell yourself to the PR office or agency as much as to any editor, so don't forget to show impressive samples of your work and a strong profile.

Chapter 13

Finding inspiration from everyday life

Do you ever find it hard to stay inspired and come up with strong ideas? If so, you're not alone – many writers struggle with inspiration – but help is at hand. When I'm feeling uninspired, I turn to online resources, social groups, and personal experiences in my everyday life to turn a blank screen into an inspired piece of writing, and critically, into a sale.

Keep up with local news

Your local newspaper may seem full of mediocrity, but sometimes local news can help you find just the story that you need to secure a commission with a national publication. Get yourself onto mailing lists for your local neighbourhood watch, police news, and local press highlights. I live in a small town in Buckinghamshire and receive our local police newsletter regularly. A recent report inside, said that Thames Valley Police had stopped a number of elderly people who had been driving on expired licences. This formed the basis of an article on road safety among senior drivers, which I sold to *Good Motoring* magazine.

Health often comes up in the local newspaper – a child sent to America for cancer treatment made it into my local paper recently. People raised £250,000 to fund his treatment and it saved his life. That kind of story would have national appeal too, so if there's a health story that you could diplomatically cover in the national press, it may present a good opportunity. Sometimes people are seeking publicity to help them raise funds for the treatment, so would be more than willing to cooperate. Where fund-raising is concerned, it's usually easy to find their contact details too.

Think how you could use local news in all areas of your writing. If you ever dabble in fiction, you might get inspired by a real-life story. Our local newspaper reported that the council was trying to evict a young man living in a tent in the woods near High Wycombe. The young man said that since he'd been living in the wild, he'd never been healthier. A media circus ensued, including a television documentary about the 'eviction'. There's plenty to draw upon from a story like this, especially if you can get an interview.

Be aware of special dates and anniversaries

Calendars of upcoming dates are an excellent source of inspiration. All magazines need suitable articles for the big events like Valentine's Day and Christmas, but also think about Shrove Tuesday, St George's Day, and some of the lesser known events like Tinnitus Awareness Week. These can provides hooks for some good stories, especially in the food and health sector where you can create special pancake fillings for readers to enjoy on Pancake Day, or a medieval banquet for St George's Day.

Smaller annual events (Pancake Day, rather than Christmas) also means your idea is less likely to be one of hundreds fighting for the same themed slot. Online calendars serve as a useful reminder of these special occasions.

These sorts of themes work really well in food and cookery publications because you can have chocolate indulgence recipes for Valentine's Day and Easter, or for health publications, a recipe for some healthy chocolate treats. You could write a review of the antioxidant benefits of high cocoa content dark chocolate, or conjure up some fruity salads for World Heart Day. With a little imagination it can be quite easy to create a recipe that fits the theme.

Keep an eye on anniversaries coming up and don't forget the gardening market for these themed foodie topics. I've sold articles for World Heart Day to gardening magazines, outlining

the benefits of home-grown produce on cardiovascular health.
www.bankholidaydates.co.uk/GreatBritain
www.nhslocal.nhs.uk/my-health/equip/events/list

Turn experiences into a sale

Look at everything you do as a potential article. When you visit a stately home, is there an angle that would be of interest to a gardening magazine? When you visit your doctor's surgery for health checks or screening, is there an angle you could sell to a health magazine? When you visit a restaurant, is there potential to sell a review to a foodie magazine?

I rarely visit an open garden these days without my camera and an open mind, looking for article opportunities and a new angle that might appeal to a gardening magazine. Not much passes me by without consideration of its story potential.

Make the most of online resources

There are many online resources which can provide inspiration for the aspiring writer. Every morning I sit down to check my Facebook, Twitter, and Science Daily alerts, all of which provide hooks and inspiration for feature ideas. Today, the strongest idea is 'Does Sugar Make You Stupid?' It's come through a news link outlining a study which shows that a high sugar diet reduces memory and intelligence amongst mice – and by implication, in humans. This could form the basis of a discussion piece on sugar in a health publication perhaps?

Join groups and meet people

When you're looking for true life stories to cover, it can be very helpful to get out and meet people. I met an old friend that I hadn't seen in 20 years at a hen party. She had Chronic Fatigue Syndrome and mercury toxicity from inhaling mercury amalgam during her years spent working as a dental nurse. I wrote her story up for a woman's magazine, then sold a similar piece to another publication.

I sold an article to a Christian publication about a local pastor who used a caravan to engage with troubled teenagers on the streets. I only found out about the caravan after going to a local church event where the pleasing results of this unusual style of outreach were presented.

Recently, when I heard that a new television series of 'Call the Midwife' was scheduled, I secured a commission with a women's magazine to write an article interviewing a 1940s midwife about her experiences and linking it to the television programme. This was only possible because I'd been out and met people with stories to tell, one of whom just happened to be a midwife in the 1940s.

You could speak to anyone working in a gardening role, health occupation, or within the food industry and uncover interesting stories about their occupation, experiences, and quirks of the job. Most people have an interesting story to tell if you only ask the right questions.

Joining a writing group can be quite valuable for making friends with the same interests and getting feedback on your work. You will also meet other people with all sorts of interesting stories and learn from each other's writing experiences.

Make the most of your pets (and other people's)!

Keeping guinea pigs has enabled me to sell photographs of my pets to various women's magazines and to write about them for a variety of animal publications in both the adult and children's markets. My guinea pigs, Rodney and Harry, have appeared in Love It, Full House, and Woman's Weekly. After a visit to the vet, I learnt that one of them was allergic to his bedding – I'm sure there's an article in that story somewhere!

I have covered guinea pig health too – looking at the effect of Nelson's Rescue Remedy for Pets on my wimpy guinea pig, Rodney. That was a fun one to write.

I've also engaged with other animal owners to write about hearing dogs for deaf people, and the therapeutic value of connecting with a dancing dog for children with disabilities.

Take a look at freelance job boards

There are websites, like Elance or Guru, dedicated to offering freelance job opportunities. You can sign up to these sites for free, search for opportunities in freelance writing and bid for the job if you see something you like. I haven't spent a lot of time on it, but I have heard that there are some good opportunities if you have time to browse and you're selective about what you bid for. Having said that, there are a lot of very badly paid jobs advertised, and you can waste a lot of time on it. Proceed with caution. www.elance.com

Develop your portfolio

If you're new to writing, then you'll need a portfolio of work to show potential customers and one way to get a portfolio is to do some work for free. Magazines who don't pay writers are often more responsive than those who pay, and this means they are in a position to help you create a portfolio of published work which will hopefully lead to better things.

Among the many non-paying health magazines in the UK are *Simply Beautiful, OM Yoga and Lifestyle,* and *Health Store Magazine.* This is just the tip of the iceberg. Look for small local publications, freebees, and very niche titles that sell in low volumes.

Read magazines

I was completely uninspired when it came to pitching Christmas feature ideas when I started freelance writing full-time. The result was, I didn't get much published that December! So the following spring, I decided to prepare early and sat down in the garden with an old Christmas copy of Prima. I read through their articles and readers letters, then without breaching anyone's copyright, I developed a wealth of my own ideas for the Christmas season that year, inspired by some of the themes they had covered the year earlier – shopping, cooking, presents and in-laws! I worked up some of my own angles on these topics and I had much better sales for that December.

Recent copies of magazines also show you what they are publishing now, and reading recent issues can provide inspiration for features, either for the magazine in hand, or indeed, for other publications!

Exercise

Flick through a local newspaper and create a list of ideas for the health, food, and gardening markets based on what you read. Is there a new restaurant opening, a new garden opening to the public, or someone with a horticulture business that's got an interesting tale to tell? Perhaps there is someone with a fascinating health condition that you'd like to cover? Or someone who conquered cancer against all odds? Look at the adverts as well as the editorial, and jot down ideas for stories.

Chapter 14

The myths of freelance writing

Freelance writing is surrounded by myths and misconceptions. Many people envisage impossible barriers to success and give up at the first sign of an obstacle. Some people never submit their work, or are left disillusioned, and riddled with self-doubt, after taking too much notice of negative people who don't share their vision. In this chapter, I'll unveil some of the most common myths of freelance writing.

Myth 1: You won't succeed. It's too competitive

Freelance writing is *not* too competitive for someone who is prepared to put the work in to hone their craft and work the hours necessary, to build any new business. Don't expect great pay for the first year (or possibly two) but this improves as you build contacts, and as editors start to have faith in your work.

Anything that's enjoyable is competitive. Marketing is competitive, design is competitive, performing arts is competitive. The better jobs in cookery, healthcare and gardening can be competitive too! Like any other occupation, as a freelance writer you usually have to start at the bottom unless you have great contacts, or a spark of pure brilliance and a lot of luck.

Most writers work up their reputation and portfolio to achieve bigger and better things as each year passes. That's what I did with my early marketing career before I got into publishing, and that's what I'm doing now with my writing career. Neither is too competitive – unless you're prone to giving up easily – and then I guess a lot of things are too competitive.

Myth 2: You need life experience first

I'd disagree – although I admit life experience helps. There is no reason why a child with a good imagination can't concoct a perfectly publishable work of fiction – that's the beauty of fiction – some of it is so out of this world that you don't have to know anything about anything (except how to write a decent story) to succeed. It completely depends on the tale. Some fiction does require a lot of research and life experience is helpful. Other fiction doesn't.

As for non-fiction, don't let anyone tell you that you can't succeed just because you're young. Write about what you know – school, music, holidays, relationships, teenage angst, interviews – or food and gardening perhaps? If your school offers horticulture experiences at a stately home, who's to say that a gardening magazine wouldn't be interested in hearing a child's perspective on these things? I honestly think that could go down a treat!

What about debates on the health credentials of your school meals? Teen magazines want youthful perspectives on all sorts of topics. If it's well argued and articulately put, a young person's perspective on other hot topics could appeal to older readers too. Being young can be a selling point if you are a good writer and you're able to communicate in an easy-to-read and upbeat fashion. I've recently spotted articles written specifically by young people in *Families First* and *Good Motoring* magazine. The selling point on each of these articles, was that they offered a young person's perspective on an adult issue.

Myth 3: You should never pitch an idea to more than one publication

Following this rule, which crops up in a lot of writing books and on courses, was a big mistake, I believe, when I was trying to make it as a writer in my youth. Back in the 1990s, writers were expected to send a query letter by Royal Mail and then wait months for a reply! Today I have bills to pay! When I became a successful freelance writer, not only did I have the benefit of the internet which made querying faster, cheaper, and much more efficient, but I threw this ridiculous rule out of the window, and pitched to everyone incessantly until someone said yes. If two editors come back wanting the same story – and they did – then you have a number of options. Either suggest something slightly different to the second publication – you mustn't sell exactly the same piece twice – or if the query is open to a degree of interpretation (as mine was) write your article twice from two different angles. Mine was on health benefits of garden produce. So when I received two identical commissions from different publications within ten minutes of one another, I accepted both and covered the topic looking at different vegetables, and different research studies for each publication.

The bottom line is that editors don't generally respond to queries from unknown freelancers unless they want to commission your article. If however, you are a known contributor to the publication, you might want to give them first refusal and wait for a response. If they know you, they are usually much more responsive. At the start of your career however, most of your queries will seem to fall on deaf ears. You can't be sitting around waiting months for that evasive reply if you need to work. Once you have made contact with an editor, by all means, be polite and give them first refusal, but don't let this rule stop your career in its tracks before you've even got started.

Myth 4: You can't possibly write for the big names until you're well known

This is simply not true. If you are a good writer, there is no reason why you can't kick start your career writing for big names and glossy magazines. I know someone whose first article was published in Cosmopolitan. However, the glossies are more difficult to break into than some of the smaller magazines and niche publications, so don't limit your aspirations to them. You might find your best early opportunities lie in writing for the free give-away magazines at your local health shop, or for your local horticultural society magazine.

Myth 5: You need a journalism qualification to be a journalist

I am a successful freelance journalist, and I don't have a journalism qualification. When I was 16 I had a meeting with the editor of the local newspaper, who told me to get A-levels, and when I'd done that, he told me to get a journalism degree. But they didn't offer the subject locally, and I didn't have the funds or inclination for a lifetime of debt, so I studied psychology locally instead. I do feel that was a decision of dubious wisdom, but I made it as a writer eventually, without journalism qualifications. I've even heard that many journalism graduates fail to get employment in the industry, so I'm inclined to think that success is more about writing ability and specialist knowledge, accompanied by the drive and tenacity to succeed, than it is about qualifications.

A journalism qualification might help you get a staff job, but don't let the absence of qualifications put you off freelancing. I am also of the belief that it is more difficult sometimes to get work with the local press than the national press. Don't let the small minds of local newspapers make you think that you can't succeed at a higher level. My article proposals still get dismissed by the local press, even though I am working for magazines across the world.

Myth 6: You need to study the magazine before pitching

Studying the magazine before pitching your article idea certainly helps, and some magazines have a very distinct style, which you couldn't hope to emulate without seeing a copy. However, I have written articles for magazines I've never seen before, notably overseas magazines and ones that I couldn't get a copy of, for whatever reason. I have also pitched ideas, and then asked the editor to send me a copy of the magazine when the idea was accepted, to enable me to get the style right. I wouldn't recommend this generally, as they do expect you to be familiar with their magazine, but if you can't get hold of one, it's either ask, order it online, or call their advertising department and pretend to be a potential advertiser! If all else fails, or you just don't have the nerve, look up their website to get a feel for the style of the publication. I've done this before, and succeeded. I've even had editors in the USA send me examples of previous articles to show the style they require for my particular piece of work.

Myth 7: The editor's decision is final

When one editor told me to go away and read the magazine, I explained that I had! I'd written my query relating exactly to what was in the latest edition, and humorously showed him just how close it was. He agreed that I'd made a good point, and the latest edition was perhaps not fully reflective of their usual approach. However, he changed his mind about rejecting my ideas and gave me a commission, followed by another and then another. In fact, I have been working for him for almost two years now!

That said, don't presume that you can always change an editor's mind. If you persistently try you could become very annoying and alienate them. Only double check if the editor's reason for rejection is clearly a bit bonkers, or perhaps you think that he hasn't understood something.

Myth 8: You must use double line spacing

When I started writing professionally in 2011, I was worried about all sorts of things that I don't even think about now. Questions like 'should I submit my article as a double or single spaced document?' The question seemed so basic and so simple, yet no one on any online forum seemed to know the answer! In the interests of getting on with it, I had to make a decision. I figured that in the digital age, the old requirement for double spacing was redundant – that was for the days when you sent hard copies in the post and the editorial team edited your work by hand. Some publications still do that, and specify it on their contributor guidelines, but today, most publications work in the modern digital world.

I've heard different and opposing arguments on the topic and it seems to me that old-fashioned people (both editors and writers) seem to like double line spacing, and those people who recognise that the world has moved into a digital age, prefer single spacing. I just send everything in single spacing by email, unless the publication guidelines explicitly dictate otherwise. So far, no one's complained, so I guess I'm doing it right.

I think mostly, it doesn't matter. I know another writer who submits everything in 1½ line spacing. As long as your work is tidy and void of errors, they probably don't care. If they have the document electronically, they can easily change it to any format they like.

Myth 9: Never write long queries/short queries

For most magazines in the UK, a couple of paragraphs are usually sufficient for a query, as editors don't have the time or inclination to read queries that are longer than that. However, I do know some editors in the UK who like the query to be almost as long as the article – then if they like it, your task is essentially a honing job, perfecting the content of your very long query.

In the USA, it's a different world. Queries can be two pages long – although one page is more usual. However, it's not essential to follow these guidelines either. My queries to the United States are usually about two paragraphs long and it still works for me. There are no rules – just find out what the editor likes and write your query emails accordingly.

Myth 10: You must submit speculatively to build a portfolio

Some people think you need to write 'on spec' to build your portfolio and increase your workload, but I don't agree. I started off in the 1990s writing articles on spec. It didn't work. Even now, with years behind me and an impressive client list, I don't sell much sent 'on spec' – not without getting the go-head and intention to buy from the editor first anyway.

You are much more likely to succeed if an editor first expresses an interest in the topic with a view to accepting it – assuming you don't mess up the actual production of the article in the intervening period. I have found that items written with prior agreement, are rarely rejected. They are not the same as a firm commission – they are still accepted on sight of the completed article, rather than commissioned on faith. But a topic the editor is interested in, anticipating, and has scheduled space for in his magazine, is always going to have more chance of success than a finished article, sent completely cold, to an editor who has no space in the foreseeable future!

Myth 11: Editors are gods

Editors are humans with all the annoying habits that the rest of us acquire. They'll give you a poor brief, edit your work so that the final copy in print is just plain wrong, and they'll mess you around from time to time – but most of these things are forgivable.

However, beware of editors who will happily waste your time, sending you off to complete a project 'on spec' that they subsequently reject for no good reason, and those who'll give you an errand to obtain photos from overseas companies only to turn down the article when you finally acquire the shots.

I encountered one editor years ago, who sent me off to complete an article on stress and nutrition, then rejected it, saying she'd had other ideas on how I might approach the topic, but had failed to tell me what they were. She added that it wasn't worth discussing the ideas in her head now, because my article was far from ideal. The point at which the editor expects you to be a mind reader is the time to move on.

I had another experience quite recently with an editor who tasked me with securing photographs from Hollywood in order to secure a commission. I was phoning America regularly chasing these photos, on the promise of a feature, and when I finally managed to secure the relevant photographs, he just seemed to have lost interest altogether. He kept making excuses and the commission never came. The time-sensitive feature idea gradually became less saleable anyway after he'd delayed and delayed.

When I encounter editors like that – people who waste your time and happily run up your phone bill on a whim, I tend to avoid them, and target editors who treat me with more respect instead. It does help if you can learn to recognise the timewasters quickly and move on.

Myth 12: Writing for free is bad news

Sometimes it is worth either writing, or letting people reprint your published work for free if you stand to benefit from it. You might benefit from either the exposure, or from something else they are able to offer – like their help with another article. I recently provided an article to the editor of a local magazine in exchange for using some of his photographs in a different article. We did each other a favour and both benefited without any money changing hands. I got paid for the article that used his photos, and he got paid for producing the magazine that contained my article. It's worth having a few contacts like this. Ignore anyone who says you should never write for free. Sometimes there might be a good reason why you should write for free. I made $500 from that article and I couldn't have sold it without his pictures.

Myth 13: When something is rejected you've wasted all that time

Material is rarely wasted. The nature of writing for a living means you will probably always have surplus material which has never made it into print. This material can form the basis for new ideas and new angles.

Many writers like to take a notebook everywhere to capture moments of inspiration in the most unusual circumstances. This makes sense – for me, these moments of inspiration come in the middle of the night when I can't sleep. My notepad comes in very handy! Jot everything down, or you'll forget those gems of inspiration. You'll probably also find that writing down the thoughts running through your head in the middle of the night will help to quieten your mind so that you can get some sleep!

Myth 14: Never pitch too early

How far in advance should you pitch an idea? British magazines vary in their lead times, but many monthly publications work four to six months ahead, others work up to a year ahead. Weeklies tend to have shorter lead times than monthlies. You'll start to get a feel for lead times with each publication you work for. In the UK markets, I usually pitch four to six months ahead of any critical date or event. There are no hard and fast rules on when to pitch. I did have one British editor who thought I was being ridiculous suggesting an idea for publication in six months' time, but for most publications, that's a good time to get your ideas in. Magazines in the USA typically have longer lead times of around six to nine months, so I have to think even further ahead when pitching time/date critical articles to the States.

Exercise

Consider the limitations which you think are holding you back in your writing career. Are they self-imposed limitations? Are you believing myths and obeying unhelpful rules that are preventing you from getting more writing commissions and realising your dream? Challenge your assumptions and consider whether the rules you are working to are really valid, or whether they are holding you back. Is there something in your approach that needs to change? Don't be so radical that you alienate editors, but do think this through. Write down what rules you are working to, and consider which, if any, might be holding you back.

Chapter 15

Unfortunate truths

Truth 1: Speculative submissions can be a headache

I have experienced some instances when the editors who only accept articles 'on spec' can be a bit of a headache. They might express an interest in your idea, sending you away to write it up, but then they don't seem to place much value on the work and are quick to reject it, saying it wasn't what they had in mind. Why they don't tell you what they have in mind at the start is anyone's guess.

I was asked to submit a completed piece of work to a local publication, after I'd become established. I did it purely as a good will gesture in support of the publication, not because I needed to build my portfolio or had anything to gain from it. The editor had shown an interest in the topic, so it wasn't completely cold, but he didn't use the piece and didn't even bother to reply until months later, when I mentioned it and he just said, "Oh yes... sorry."

It wasn't a bad piece of work. It formed the basis of another article which I sold to a paying publication later in the year.

I've also had editors ask me to write an article only to declare that they've had 'second thoughts' on the subject matter after it's been submitted. If an editor is not fully committed to commissioning a piece of work, then don't spend hours and hours perfecting it, unless you're prepared to take the fall.

On the upside, when you take a risk and it does all go wrong, you can often find an alternative buyer for your work, as I did in the example given.

Truth 2: You need six months to break into the market

With freelance writers mostly being paid on publication, there can be long delays in getting paid. If you quit your job to write full-time, you need sufficient savings, or support from a partner, to get you through six months of full-time working without pay.

It usually takes at least six months to build up your network of contacts, get a few commissions, and critically, start getting paid. This six month period of grace gives you the time to break into the freelance writing market, without having to worry about mounting bills and rent arrears. By the end of that period, if you're any good at it, you should find the money is starting to trickle in. However, it could be a long time before you're earning your full market worth.

Truth 3: Payment on publication can take years

It's good to have a decent financial cushion to fall back on, even after your six month 'getting started' period, because some publications take years to pay. If they pay on publication, and keep putting your article back, especially with a monthly or quarterly title, it can easily slip back months, or even years. I've had articles written two years ago, which were accepted but have not been published yet. Fortunately, that publication paid on acceptance, but there's one other article, written for a different publication almost two years ago, that is still in the pipeline, awaiting its place in the publishing schedule. For that piece, I haven't yet been paid, although I am assured we'll get there eventually!

It's also worth noting that if your item isn't scheduled, not all publishers will tell you when it's out. If you miss it, and you don't invoice, you may not get paid, so it's well worth keeping an eye out when you know something is scheduled. I almost missed a piece which was published recently, only discovering that it had been published because it came up on a web search under my name. I invoiced the magazine and they said, 'Oh yes, it was published in the print edition months ago!' I hadn't invoiced, and it appears that they weren't going to pay me unless I did. You need to keep your finger on the pulse of what's going in when, and keep on top of your invoicing.

Truth 4: You might need to write for free to develop a portfolio

If you are having trouble getting a portfolio together, one way to get started is to be willing to write for free. There are lots of small press publications who are looking for material but can't afford to pay. Some of them might be a headache to work with but fortunately you don't need a huge portfolio.

I started freelance writing with three published items on nutrition to my name. I'd written them for free to promote my nutrition consultancy some years earlier, then when I started writing for a living, these three articles provided the foundations of my growing portfolio of published work.

So the truth is, this isn't an easy industry, but for those who see writing as a vocation, not just as a job, the downsides are no big hardship. The upsides of having the freedom to choose what work you do, and to choose what hours you work, far outweigh the challenges.

Exercise

Do you have a portfolio of work already? If not, write down your specialist subjects and identify which local or niche magazines could help get you into print. Then contact the editor and run a few ideas past them. If they say they'd like you to write an article on a topic you've discussed, even if they don't pay for contributions, why not oblige? You still get examples for your portfolio – along with a sense of satisfaction from seeing your work in print.

Chapter 16

Lessons from frustrating editorial communications

Editorial communications can be very frustrating. They are such busy people that I'm sure many of my email communications are completely overlooked! Here are some of the lessons I've learnt from frustrating editorial communications.

When the editor goes deadly quiet

Last year I received an email response from a magazine editor saying "Yes I like the idea of this, so would be happy to commission. I'll send you over one of our model contracts shortly"... but the model contract never arrived. I chased up a couple of times, and in good faith, I began working on the article – fully aware that previously, he'd told me to never start work on an article until I receive the contract. But I was having a slow period and had confidence that the contract would follow shortly. It didn't. Unable to get a response by email, I left it another few weeks, and then telephoned and left messages, but neither emails nor telephone messages were ever responded to.

Three months' later, the subject matter was dating, and another magazine had shown interest in the idea... but they only paid one eighth of the fee. I really wanted to sell the article to the first editor but couldn't get hold of him! I thought he'd just changed his mind. Can I write it twice I wondered? Having worked for the first magazine before, I knew their model contract forbids this, but then, I hadn't received it yet!

I started to wonder if I was out of favour, or if he was ill, dead or left the company. I tried his deputy and still couldn't get a response. I phoned again expecting voicemail, and nearly fell off my chair when the editor picked up the phone and told me he still wanted to proceed. I was on his list, but he'd just been really busy. Phew! So I waited.

Another month passed. I pinged a few more ideas by email just to stay in touch and see if he liked anything. No response. I tried phoning again and got his answerphone. I left a message but received no response.

I never received the contract and I'd written the article but couldn't get anyone on the editorial team to acknowledge my communications.

I sold the article to the magazine which didn't pay so well in the end – before the subject matter was out of date. The cheeky part of me thinks I should have just sent it in, but if they'd overlooked it – as they did with the rest of my emails – I wouldn't have been paid at all.

What I learnt:

- Being scared of the telephone is not an option. It really is an essential tool for communicating with those editors who just don't respond to emails.
- Sometimes, you just can't win. As a freelancer, it's easy to let your imagination get carried away wondering why a certain editor hasn't responded. You just need to have a thick skin and move on. After all, if they don't respond, they can't be that keen, and you still have bills to pay, so try elsewhere!
- Be aware that when you're starting to draft an article without a contract (when one is expected) you may end up falling flat on your face without a sale.

When the editor forgets to commission

On another occasion, I received an email from a niche newspaper apologising that they would have to put back publication of my article because of other priorities.

"What article?" I had to ask, as I knew nothing of this

commission! It transpires that they wanted me to write a feature on stress which I'd pitched to them months earlier but no one had responded to tell me.

So I phoned the editor to find out the fee, word count, and deadline – then I accepted the commission. I submitted the feature by email a week or so later, asking if they needed a picture of my interviewee, and whether I could invoice them. They didn't reply so I sent the invoice anyway. The article duly appeared in the newspaper, but their communications didn't extend to the accounts department and I had to chase up the invoice later, which had, apparently, been deleted!

What I learnt:

- The importance of following up pitches cannot be under-estimated, as I almost missed out on the commission for the article on stress management because the newspaper thought they'd already commissioned it, and they hadn't.
- Do keep on top of your invoicing and what's been paid – otherwise you might not get paid.

When payment is long overdue

On the subject of getting paid, I once held one of my scheduled articles to ransom with a publisher who owed me payment for four features already, and one of the invoices was 4 months overdue. I was starting to wonder if they were about to go bust. The tactic worked and I received payment for all four articles by the end of the week. I've written another four articles for them since then, and remarkably perhaps, the payment schedule has improved!

What I learnt:

- Don't be afraid of being a pest when payments are overdue. There's a balance to be struck between tolerance of slow payers who you want to keep sweet, and just letting them get away without paying you at all! Keep on top of your invoicing and if you have to hold your next article to ransom, it's a strategy that I have found works.

When they use your work without telling you

One publication that only accepts articles on spec, is proving to be particularly challenging. They originally contacted me about an article I'd submitted because they wanted it tweaked. I duly complied and resubmitted it. The piece was accepted for publication, and I was told it would be many months before they had space to publish it.

Five months' later I was searching my name on Google and this article came up. It had been published after just 2 months and no one had mentioned it, or importantly, paid me. If they hadn't put it online, I'd never have known. I queried with the editor how a writer is supposed to know when to invoice if they don't tell them when their contribution is published, and she said she expected all her writers to be subscribers. Hmmm.

That was three months ago, and I invoiced them promptly. They still haven't paid. I am chasing monthly and getting the distinct impression that they don't want to pay me.

At that same time, I asked the editor if she would be interested in another article, and she said yes, she'd like to see it on spec. I sent it over by return, as it was a reprint. I never heard any more, until I chased it up a month later and she said she intended to print it towards the end of the year.

If I hadn't chased her about it, I may have never known it had been accepted, and importantly, I wouldn't have known that I needed to invoice them for payment in due course.

The whole experience leaves me wondering which of the other numerous 'on spec' articles, submitted in the early days of my writing career, they actually printed (and for which I have never been paid). I asked the question and she didn't know.

What I learnt:

- If you send an article 'on spec' always chase for a rejection or acceptance.
- If it's accepted, always keep an eye out in forthcoming publications to see if it's made it into print. When you spot it, invoice promptly.
- Don't rely on publishers to pay you. Be proactive in chasing your dues.

Chapter 17

Writing for online markets

There is a growing trend for people to read online, rather than buy printed publications, and that trend has created a growing market for writers of online materials. Whether they are e-magazines, blogs, or news and lifestyle websites, there are many opportunities in this sector. It has an almost insatiable demand for new words and material daily. However, by the nature of the internet, most information is free and so payment can be poor or non-existent. However, developing a name for yourself as a blogger can get you a following, which may in turn, make it easier for you to gain paid work, and secure a book contract if you have ambitions that way. Many websites are funded by advertising, so that could also be a source of revenue. You can monetise your blog by activating Google AdSense, which runs adverts on your blog, if you wish.

The range of e-magazines available online is constantly growing as traditional publishing moves to online publishing as a cheaper alternative, potentially, with a wider, international audience.

The glossy British lifestyle magazine, *Easy Living*, has recently declared that it is going online and ceasing publication of its printed edition. It's one of many that have gone online during the economic downturn.

Online publishing is growing while the print-based magazine industry shrinks in these tough economic times. That's why opportunities in online markets are not to be overlooked.

Writing for the internet can be quite different to writing for print publications. There is a tendency online for people to want short, punchy information that gets straight to the point. Readers are less interested in some of the chatty material published in print magazines. Those who are seeking more information will click on hyperlinks in the text to pages offering more detail. This approach is particularly common on health websites where one symptom or diagnosis links to another, and the range of alternative therapies for any given complaint may each have a page of their own.

A wide range of e-magazines is shown at www.onlinemagazineshub.com. This site lists e-magazines published from all around the world. They cover diverse categories from agriculture to politics; to home and garden, to science and technology. There are food, cooking, health and fitness categories too! You can search by category, or by language, and if you're a multilingual writer, then opportunities abound!

Many magazines have their contributor guidelines available on their website. The guidelines detail what kinds of materials they are interested in, their terms and rates of pay. It's worth checking for guidelines online before you contact the editor of your chosen publication, regardless of whether it's web-based or in print.

There are also many opportunities to write for online blogs, and a good example here is the Guardian newspaper's blog, www.guardian.co.uk/tone/blog. They cover all sorts of material from green living, to allotments and gardening, to camera clubs.

Mslexia has a blog for female writers and they actively encourage applications from people wanting to write their blog for a three month period. Visit www.mslexia.co.uk for more information. Blogging sites like Suite 101 or Love to Know also offer a variety of blogging opportunities enabling writers to cover the subjects that interest them – although the pay on many of these opportunities may be less than fantastic.

Remember that people browsing the web tend to have a shorter attention span and are looking for instant information and quick snippets, not necessarily detailed discussions. It is possible to draw people into discussions online, but you need to get to the point very quickly or you've lost them.

The web is information-rich, but the people using it are time-poor. They need quick answers and the amount of information can be overwhelming. If the page they open doesn't meet their needs at a glance, they won't spend any further time on it.

Lots of bullets can be helpful to break up the text. Pictures and diagrams make your article easier to digest. Snippets of information work well when writing for the online market. Then you can perhaps add links to additional information if they want to read about the topic in more detail.

Exercise

Go onto Google or your favourite search engine, and search for a gardener's blog, food blog, or a health blog, relating to your key area of interest. You'll find The Guardian blogs, BBC blogs and many other blogs come up. Peruse them for opportunities to contribute, and maybe you'll get inspiration for a blog of your own.

Chapter 18

Writing a book

While article writing always challenges you to get the most information into the smallest possible space, writing a book is a completely different ball game. You have so much more space to fill, that you are able to go into greater detail. You are no longer constrained by word count limitations to the same extent, but you have to hold the reader's attention for much longer. You can discuss your deepest thoughts, most complex gardening strategies, most annoying health frustrations, and strangest food delicacies in greater detail.

When you've been writing articles for a living, typically limited to 1000 words, it's an indulgence to write a book. But it's also a challenge to break the habit of a lifetime and write in-depth, covering all that detail that your magazine articles just never had space to cover!

The market for books is diverse but what most publishers want is a title that has mass market appeal, so that it will sell in its thousands, preferably millions, all around the world. Isn't that what everyone wants? Yes, of course it is, but the unfortunate fact of the matter is, if you're not a well-known personality, then it can be pretty difficult even to get an agent, let alone to get a book deal! Celebrity faces help sell books – but most unknown authors seeking their first book deal, struggle.

Many of the bigger publishing houses are no longer willing to deal with authors directly, and will only deal with agents. So you have two choices – either you single out those publishers who deal with authors directly, or you get an agent. Look at the publishers who are printing books on the kinds of subjects that you want to cover. Contact some of them directly and they'll soon tell you whether they accept proposals and manuscripts directly from authors, or whether they only deal with agents.

To find an agent, The Writers' and Artists' Yearbook in the UK, The Australian Writer's Marketplace, or The Writers Market in the USA, are excellent resources. They each contain a complete listing of agents and their specialist topics. In some cases, they provide details of the authors on their books, and their fees.

If you do decide to approach a publisher directly, then the usual rule of thumb is to provide a synopsis of your proposed book, including a chapter breakdown, and the first completed chapter as a taster of what is to come. It can takes months for publishers to respond to proposals, so you need to be patient, but don't be put off if one publisher turns you down. It often takes multiple attempts to get an idea accepted. Most best-selling authors have suffered rejection, but they are famous now because they didn't give up, and eventually they got the break they needed.

There are a few publishers who have schemes specifically for new writers. One such publisher is Harper Collins whose site, www.authonomy.com, enables writers to upload their manuscripts. Visitors to the website then read, comment on, and rank each contribution, and if your book gets good feedback Harper Collins will look at it with a view to possibly offering you a contract.

Until fairly recently, Pan MacMillan welcomed manuscripts to its 'MacMillan New Writing Scheme'. At the time of writing the imprint is closed to new submissions, but it's worth keeping an eye on their website in case it opens again:

www.panmacmillan.com/Imprints

It's worth mentioning at this point, that there is another straight forward approach – John Hunt Publishing (JHP), the publisher behind Compass Books – who published this book – have imprints that deal with a range of other niche titles.

One of their imprints, Ayni Books, specialises in alternative health, and another JHP imprint, Moon Books, specialises in paganism and shamanism, relevant for those authors wishing to write about spiritual or traditional approaches to health... or perhaps developing a more spiritual garden atmosphere!

John Hunt Publishing has a very streamlined and efficient approach. They are quick to respond to ideas and proposals, and it's delightful to receive a book contract quickly – although suddenly having a huge amount of work to do might seem daunting!

On the plus side, John Hunt Publishing deals directly with authors (so you don't need an agent) and is willing to take on niche titles that may not have mass-market appeal.

On the minus side, because they are a small publisher, they are unable to pay advances, so you have to wait for the royalties to roll in. Depending on what contract you are offered, there may be a financial contribution to make on your part, although for the first two levels of contract, this doesn't apply.

There are four different levels of contract available from John Hunt publishing. I was offered level two. They offer different contracts to different authors depending on how well they think your book will sell and how well known you are. It's worth reading through the contracts properly if you get an idea accepted in principle, as depending on which contract you are offered, you may, or may not, find the terms acceptable to you.

To submit your health book idea to Ayni Books or Moon Books, the process is simple – just visit the relevant website below and follow the instructions.

www.ayni-books.com/jhp-get-published.html

www.moon-books.net/jhp-get-published.html

To see the full range of imprints visit www.johnhuntpub-lishing.com/our-imprints.html

If all else fails, there is always self-publishing. Self-publishing using Amazon's online tool to convert your word document into an e-book is a straightforward process and you get a good cut of the selling price which Amazon makes clear, as you go through the process. At the time of writing, it's 70%.

If you want your book self-published in print, then it's worth checking ads in writing magazines, for publishers who will publish your work for a fee. Be warned though, that some of these services can be very expensive, and the vanity publishing industry has gained a bad reputation over the years. Not to say that there haven't been self-published successes – there have – but they are few and far between. There's nothing like having a real publishing house behind you with all their distribution networks and valuable contacts, especially if you want to be published in a tangible book made of paper, and distributed around the world!

Exercise

Write a synopsis and chapter breakdown for your best book idea. Perhaps you're not ready to approach a publisher yet, but this helps to get your ideas straight, and you can see where the gaps exist and add to it over time. When you're ready to submit your proposal to a publisher, it's a good idea to write the first chapter too, and submit it with your completed proposal.

Chapter 19

Putting the finishing touches to your work

One thing that I have learnt over the years is never to submit your work in too much of a hurry. It is so easy, when you've been working on a piece of writing, to not notice the small but significant errors in the text. Don't rely on the editors to tidy it up for you. They won't be impressed to see work littered with errors. Just wait. Bide your time, and look at it again after a break, or get someone else to read it for you. You will see things that you didn't see before – not necessarily errors, but perhaps sentences that might flow better if you rephrased them, or words that you have repeated too many times in a single paragraph.

Freelance writers do have a reputation for getting distracted and leaving their writing until close to deadline. This is a very bad strategy if you want to produce good quality work. You need to allow yourself time to review and improve your work with a fresh pair of eyes. This can take weeks.

If you want editors to come back to you time and time again, don't rush things. Give them quality, take your time, go back over it enough times to have confidence that it really is as good as it can be. Don't let that initial rush of excitement when the first draft is completed, compel you to submit it prematurely. When you look at it again 24 hours' later you might wonder what on earth you were getting excited about! I've done that before.

In my early career, I made the mistake of submitting something that I later looked at in horror, spotted a couple of errors and had to resubmit. That, frankly, is embarrassing and unprofessional – but not as bad as letting something that you know is wrong, go to print. So now I take my time proofreading and double checking everything, and I recommend that you do the same.

I have a friend on Facebook, who writes for some small press magazines. To my knowledge, she doesn't get paid for it, so perhaps she doesn't regard it with the same level of perfectionism that those of us working in the paying markets expect. But she recently boasted that she'd written two articles in a day. I got the impression she'd started them, finished them, and submitted them, all in the space of a few hours!

When I read things like that, I imagine that the articles are not very good, because it gives the impression that they've been rushed, not proofread, not checked, and not edited for optimal flow. As for research and interviews, the articles probably didn't contain any.

To give this girl due credit, she may only have written a first draft of two articles that day, which would be much more sensible – or perhaps she's a genius. But I did get the impression that she had done it in a rush and submitted them in a rush. You might get away with a few minor imperfections, but be warned that when something wrong goes into a magazine the readers just love to point it out. This happened to me once when I submitted the wrong dates for a forthcoming event. At the time of writing the article, the organisers' website was displaying the 2012 dates with no year. I thought it was the date of the upcoming event in 2013, and in good faith, put the dates into my article. I received an email from the editor after it had gone on sale. It was a copy of a letter sent by a reader, pointing out that the dates were wrong. I had to grovel and promise to double check everything from then on... which I do now, almost obsessively. It seems unnecessary much of the time, but you can guarantee that the one thing that you don't double check will be the one thing that is wrong.

On another occasion, I was tasked with writing a travel article, and including some places to stay nearby. I looked online, and selected hotels and campsites near to the location. The websites looked very nice, the locations looked open.

When the publishers came to edit the piece of work, I received an email saying that they had checked the details, and one of the campsites that I had listed, was closed permanently. Since then, I have never believed a website. People close businesses all the time, but they don't necessarily shut down their websites.

If you are covering cooking classes for a food magazine, or gardens to visit, even if you know they were open and trading quite recently, always double check that they are still open – and planning to stay that way – prior to submitting your article. Not checking your details like this, reflects very badly on you as a writer and may undermine any confidence that the editor has in your work.

To provide another example, I was writing a piece that briefly mentioned the Doctor Who exhibition in Cardiff. Fortunately on that occasion, even though I'd been there only a couple of months earlier, I double checked the opening hours only to find that in the intervening period, the Doctor Who exhibition had closed down permanently. This was back in 2012, prior to the opening of the brand-new Doctor Who exhibition which stands in Cardiff today. I pulled the Doctor Who exhibition out of the article, because there was no guarantee as to when the new exhibition would be completed, and I couldn't risk the information being incorrect.

Just because the internet says something is true, doesn't necessarily mean it is true. Always double check.

A proofreader is an invaluable resource. My husband is my proofreader – he complains that it's the worst paid job he's ever had! But he points out small missing words like 'a', that as a writer immersed in a project, your mind automatically fills in. Sometimes, you don't even see that these tiny words are missing until somebody else points out the error.

He also suggests ways that things might be better expressed, occasionally queries spellings and gets me to double check facts – all of which have been very helpful. He sometimes suggests additional comments or information which he feels should be included.

A proofreader will also look for clarity to ensure that what you are trying to say is what's coming across to the reader. If he doesn't understand a part of it he'll say so, and then you can work on the clarity of the statement. Sometimes a proofreader will also help to get the word count down if an article is too long.

Exercise

Next time you write an article and feel compelled to send it in straight away, leave it for at least 24 hours, and then read through it again carefully. Do you spot errors, things that might be better phrased, or missed opportunities to mention something significant that didn't cross your mind yesterday?

Chapter 20

Marketing yourself

Even when you're busy writing and feel you have no time to take on additional work, marketing is important. There can be such a lag between querying and getting that assignment, that you can be snowed under with work one week and twiddling your thumbs a few weeks later if you don't keep pitching ideas to editors and stay on top of your marketing. Never stop querying just because you're drowning in work. By all means, slow down a bit, but remember you're not like an employee with a guaranteed workload. If you don't market yourself, you don't work... broadly speaking.

Stay in touch with editors to stay on their radar, even if you don't have an idea to pitch to them – they might have an assignment in mind that would suit you. Once an editor starts to trust you to deliver a good article by a given deadline, he or she may approach you with an article brief that they would like written. You accept the assignment, and it saves you from having to spend enormous amounts of time pitching – which in turn enables you to spend more time working and earning. This is a great situation in which to find yourself, and it took me almost two years' freelancing to establish myself and start getting commissions without actually having to ask for them. There are some basic things you should consider in terms of marketing however, and some of these are detailed below.

Get a website

Every serious writer needs a website to showcase their work. If you don't already have one, there are many free sites offering you the tools to build your own, and get your own URL, often free of charge. A website doesn't have to be expensive or onerous. A simple site will do to get you started and it can evolve over time, just as you do.

Before you get started, it's a good idea to browse other writers' websites to get a feel for the kind of look, feel, and content that you want to display on your own website. Think about your colour scheme, navigation bar, how you want to present yourself, and what downloads you want to make available. You might want to include some of the following:

- Biography or 'About me' page;
- A list of some of your clients;
- Sample articles;
- Links to online stories that you've written;
- Links to your social media pages;
- A link to your book on Amazon;
- A list of the services that you offer;
- Testimonials from editors;
- Examples of your photography;
- Information on your PR work;
- Contact details;
- A blog;
- An image of yourself so people can see who they are dealing with;
- Images of your published works – books, magazines, newspapers;
- Links to your clients' websites.

Why not add to this list yourself and create a list of what you'd like to see on your own website?

Free websites

There are many free website building tools available online. They include:

- Yola: www.yola.com
- Webs: www.webs.com
- Weebly: www.weebly.com
- Moon Fruit: www.moonfruit.com

Some people create their website using a blogging facility like www.wordpress.com or www.blogger.com. I'd suggest you play around with them and use the one that you find most intuitive, and the easiest to use.

It can take a little bit of time to get your head around how to use the content management system (the tools that enable you to edit the site), but once you've spent some time going through the options, none of these sites are too difficult to manage.

I used Google's Get British Business Online, and it served me well. However, it has now closed to new applicants.

The problems with some of these sites are that the templates are quite rigid and what you can do with them is quite limited. These limitations drive some writers to pay professional website designers to create a more flexible site for them. But unless you have big design ideas, one of these simple sites is probably good enough to get you started. As long as your site gives you a place to showcase your work, that is the most important factor.

Social media

The other hot place to be, especially if you're trying to promote your latest book, is social media. Sites like Facebook and Twitter are addictive, thriving and free! In the consumer market – e.g. when you want to promote a book – things like prize give-aways for one lucky winner who 'likes' your page and shares your post can increase your following dramatically within hours. Perhaps you are not fully aware of the benefits of social media so I'm going to discuss some of them now.

Some people use social media for fun, frivolity and as a channel to the latest news. Others are sceptical – underwhelmed by the mediocrity, pointlessness and drudgery of it all!

Wherever you stand on the spectrum, there's no denying that social media use is seeing unprecedented growth. The fastest growing demographic of social media users is the over 40s and it's now so popular that even the elderly are engaging. Watch out for your granny on Facebook sometime soon!

Now I should confess – at first, I didn't 'get' it. I joined Facebook in 2007 and had one friend. I couldn't understand why anyone would want to have their conversations in front of an audience of 300 people (none of whom knew me). I deactivated my account a few weeks' later following a BBC news report about Facebook identity theft.

I didn't return to the scene until 2010 when I had an interview for a job as a Social Media Manager and needed a crash course in understanding what it was all about. I befriended my sisters, relatives, and anyone else willing to be my Facebook friend. Then I found a few old acquaintances online too.

My news feed started to provide insight into the lives of people I didn't see very often – some of whom I hadn't seen in years, and I started to understand the point of Facebook.

It was another year however, before I was ready to condense my thoughts into 140 characters and brave the booming world of Twitter.

Frankly, I had no interest in Twitter and couldn't understand the appeal of it, until I read an article written by Matt Britland, an educational blogger whose tweets landed him a writing assignment with The Guardian.

Matt began tweeting without really understanding the point of it all – just like me! First, he posted a few messages to friends, then he started to post his opinions on education in the UK and his following grew. Before he knew it, he had a sizeable following and when he tweeted his disapproval at Michael Gove's education policies, it was followed an hour later, by a request from The Guardian newspaper to write a blog based on his tweets.

"I spent that evening channelling my fury into a post on the subject," he said (*The Power of Twitter*, The Guardian Teacher Network, 31 March 2012). The day after the blog was published, Sky News got in touch with him asking for an interview on live television. He was starting to get quite a name for himself in the world of education and it was all from posting a few opinions on Twitter.

This article spurred me to open a Twitter account and start tweeting. To date, most of my followers are aspiring writers but there are a few features editors and magazines in there too.

The challenge for me is to be sufficiently interesting without being so controversial that I alienate people. It's quite a balancing act for someone with as many controversial opinions and ideas as me!

Building your following

Now, as a writer, it helps if you have an area of expertise, and as you're reading this book, I'm guessing it's food, cooking, health, or maybe gardening! If you start to post messages about your specialist subject, you'll gain followers interested in that subject, and then, when you have something to promote, such as a new book, you'll have a ready audience interested in your work.

One example of someone who has used social media very well to promote his work is Simon Whaley, the author of 12 non-fiction books and a prolific magazine journalist. He uses Twitter to promote his blog and promote his work. As a Writer's Bureau tutor in his spare time (what a busy man!) he has a following of aspiring writers. His blog offers hints and tips to get on in publishing – and of course, he uses social media to promote his books whenever he has one published.

Social media also provides another way for editors to follow you, stay in touch, and get to know you. Some of the editors I work with follow me on Twitter.

Give your audience what they want

The key to successful social media engagement is in identifying what your audience enjoy and value, giving them lots of it, and inviting them to be interactive and engage with you. So for example, sharing links to recipes, health articles, tips on fitness, and on growing your own vegetables, might attract a following of people interested in healthy lifestyles – the sorts of people who might buy a book that you write on the subject some day.

Competitions can also drive lots of activity and help you gain new followers. The real key is to generate so much interest that people share your posts with their friends and then your following naturally grows. The term 'going viral' is now firmly established in the English language to describe the most widely shared social media posts.

The advantage of having a growing band of followers is that when you want to promote a new book, you can lure them into your story by publishing a sample of the text, in the hope of luring them into a sale. As you can see, social media as a marketing tool can serve multiple purposes from staying in touch with editors, to promoting your newly published book.

Is it for me?

Maybe you feel a little unsure about social media, the time it takes, and how difficult it is. This approach is not for everyone, but there's no denying that social media is the biggest growing medium in marketing, with arguably the greatest potential for you to engage with your audiences successfully.

Think about it – most users stay tuned into their favourite social media platforms all day long on their smart phones, so the potential for this form of promotion to provide positive inter-action with your followers is remarkable.

The greatest strength of social media is also its greatest challenge – the open interaction and the potential for negativity sends some people running in the other direction. Fortunately, negative feedback is not generally a big problem on writers' pages.

But if you're concerned about it, there are a number of ways to manage negativity. Firstly, you can set up your Facebook page so that people's ability to comment on your posts is limited. It's also very easy to delete negative comments and block the offending individuals from posting any more.

Alternatively, if you set up a 'group' on Facebook instead of a 'page', or invite people to befriend you on your private account, you can control who is accepted and block/unfriend them if you decide you don't like them.

Twitter also enables you to set up your account so that new followers must be approved by you. You can block them from viewing your feed at any time.

Why not experiment with social media? You can close your account if it's not working for you.

Blogs

The most commonly used blogging sites are www.wordpress .com or www.blogger.com. You can promote your new blogs on your Twitter or Facebook pages.

Whether or not you want to write a blog is a very personal thing. If you have things to say on a particular subject, it can be a nice way to get them off your chest! But be aware of the Communications Act 2003 and potential for libel. Blogs are arguably best used for bright, positive communications!

What you don't want is for your blog to become a burden. Do it because you enjoy it, and if you don't enjoy it, don't do it.

I did it for a while, but felt it had little to offer over my Facebook page so I closed it down.

As for other types of social media, the message is the same – enjoy or abandon. If you enjoy it then there could be some real benefit when it comes to promoting your finished works and developing a faithful following of… dare I call them 'fans'?

If social media is not for you, then there are plenty of other ways to showcase your talents – websites, talks, book signings etc. – so have a think about the possibilities and then do what's right for you.

Other approaches to marketing (especially books)

You can engage in numerous other activities to raise your profile and market yourself and your book if you have one. I have recently joined Aylesbury College's Hall of Fame. The opportunity came at a time when I felt I could benefit from raising my profile! You can also arrange radio interviews, notify the local press that you've had a book published, do book signings, offer promotional giveaways to help you build an emailing list of potential buyers, write articles about the content of your newly published book, and circulate review copies to people who have said they are willing to review your work online.

Marketing yourself as a journalist is a more direct affair. You can't beat querying and pitching ideas to win commissions from editors. But it can't do any harm to build a wider reputation for yourself as an expert in your chosen subject. Other than that, it just makes sense to always deliver brilliant copy on time and to specification. Having a book published can also add to your credibility and may help to establish you as an expert in your chosen field. Some publications, such as Reader's Digest, are much more interested in awarding article commissions to published authors than to any random journalist.

Exercise

Examine the various social media sites detailed in this chapter, and consider how you can increase your presence on social media or online. Write a list of things you would like to achieve with your online presence, and then make some notes, like a mini e-marketing plan, on how you think you can use online resources to help you achieve your aims.

Chapter 21

Avoiding legal issues

For a detailed look at journalism law, I'd recommend buying a more in-depth book on the subject, but I can highlight a few points that you should know before you get started.

Copyright

Copyright laws state that what you write is covered by copyright automatically. You don't have to get your work registered. However, if you do end up in court disputing your copyright claim, it is worth having some way of demonstrating that you really did write the first copy of the disputed material. If proof of copyright worries you, and you want to have some kind of proof that your work is in fact, your own work, then posting a sealed copy of the manuscript to yourself by registered post, and then storing it postmarked and sealed, is one way of showing that your work was your own on that date, as postmarked. This may help you in the event of a copyright infringement claim. However, this is a suggestion that has been going around in writing circles for decades – whether it stands up in court, I have no idea. You should speak to a qualified legal representative about asserting your copyright ownership if it concerns you.

This law obviously works both ways. You must not, ever, copy somebody else's work and claim it as your own. If you do, you are setting yourself up for potentially expensive legal costs, defending yourself in court, and/or paying compensation to the injured party. Not to mention the publication you work for, who could also face the same legal challenges. Don't do it. Don't risk huge legal bills for the sake of rewriting something in your own words.

If you are using somebody else's ideas for inspiration, don't make your final piece too close to what they have written, because that can get you in trouble too. Rewrite it from your own perspective, bringing your own ideas and thoughts into the work.

The exception is when you have the other author's permission to print a part of their work and give them credit for it. It is widely accepted that quoting a couple of lines from a much larger piece of work doesn't require permission if it is properly credited, however, I wouldn't risk it. This is a grey area and I would always suggest getting permission if you want to quote somebody else's work. Here's why...

In 1978, best-selling horror novelist, James Herbert, celebrated the publication of his new novel, The Spear. But the celebrations didn't last long. He was originally inspired to write the story by Trevor Ravencroft's book, The Spear of Destiny, and he openly credited Trevor Ravenscroft's work as inspiration in his Authors Note at the front of the book. He then included some facts from Ravenscroft's book in the story.

A lawsuit ensued, with Ravenscroft demanding £25,000 for the use of what Herbert believed at the time, to be historical facts. It turned out that the 'facts' were gained by Ravencroft's personal transcendental meditation. Because these 'facts' were exclusive to Ravencroft, and not available from other research sources, Herbert was not permitted to use them without permission.

In court, Herbert was ordered to remove 13 lines from his book. The paperback edition was subsequently delayed by two years, and eventually published with the 13 lines deleted and a revised prologue. Herbert gravely wished he'd never put those lines in the book in the first place.

It's also worth knowing that quotes from a pop song can cost a fortune. The music industry thinks nothing of charging an author £1000 for repeating one line from a pop song in their literary work. Don't think you can quote lines from a song for free – you can't.

I recently wanted to quote directly from a university research paper and requested their permission to do so, but they seemed uncomfortable about it. I never got permission, so eventually I rewrote the key points in my own words. For the sake of a few lines, it simply isn't worth risking a lawsuit.

Libel

Libel is when you write something offensive or defamatory about a person or organisation. Any disparaging statement can be libelous and you could end up having to defend your actions in court, regardless of whether your statement is true or false. If you want a stress-free life as a freelance writer, avoid writing anything offensive or defamatory.

I've had to think twice, even in reporting the local police updates in my local paper. Ever since someone pointed out that if the police made a mistake and I repeated it, I could be sued for libel, I've just reported the crime and punishment, not the names of the offenders. Remember, the staff reporters on the daily newspapers may be covered by a heavy-duty insurance policy, but I'm guessing you're not.

Someone who sues you for libel doesn't have to prove damage to their reputation. If the story is deemed to be defamatory, that is sufficient. If you are libellous about an organisation the directors can sue for that too.

In your defence, you can argue that your story was true, but that's easier than proving it – and do you really want to go to court anyway? If you're uncomfortable or unsure about something, it's best just to leave it out.

Blogs

Blogs are a growing area, but no more so than Facebook and Twitter. You can't fail to have noticed the alarming number of people who have been sued for posting unpopular opinions on Twitter and Facebook.

The lesson to be learnt is not to be controversial unless you're prepared to face the consequences. If you're going to be controversial, make sure you've got insurance. At the time of writing, the latest poor person to be sued over their Twitter comment was a lady who complained of non-payment by a company that she'd been working for. The company claimed it was libel and at the time of writing is seeking damages through the courts. This was all over a £140 unpaid bill – which incidentally, has now been paid. The lady was facing the prospect of financial ruin until her case was taken on by no-win no-fee lawyers – all because of an ill-advised tweet!

Unless you're prepared for the legal onslaught, just be nice. Don't say anything that might be offensive or libellous – or if you do, get insurance first.

Professional Indemnity Insurance

Insurance companies tend to consider writing as a high risk occupation, so you can't get professional indemnity insurance cheap. You can't blame them – you could write anything in newspapers published around the world and online. Anyone could take offence at anything, and before you know it, you're in court up against some big player on a charge of libel.

The risk depends on what areas of journalism you are working in. To be honest, you're unlikely to end up in court over writing about gardening unless you make some derogatory remark about a celebrity gardener, a stately home, or say something else offensive. You're also unlikely to get sued for writing a recipe unless you have copied someone else's recipe – see copyright law above.

But for peace of mind, professional indemnity insurance is worth considering. It covers you for libel claims, copyright infringement and other risks that writers may face during their career.

Health

While you may feel that food writing is relatively low risk, health is trickier – you're taking people's lives and well-being in your hands. You don't know their background, and you don't know what medication they are on. Yet you're expected to give health advice, through the pages of a magazine, newspaper, website or book, to millions of people, possibly billions, possibly all around the world. I think writing about health carries a much higher risk of being sued. Something you suggest may cause somebody to have an adverse reaction.

You may, for example, write an article saying that grapefruits are nutritionally dense and may help to lower your cholesterol. But then someone eats grapefruit and it interferes with their body's ability to absorb their essential medication. They suffer from a bad reaction because their medication is not working properly, and they sue you for giving bad advice. Incidentally, grapefruits do interfere with all sorts of medication, and are thought by some medical bodies to worsen the symptoms of arthritis.

To provide another example, let's say you write that the lycopene in tomatoes is good for a healthy heart. A reader eats lots of tomatoes, only to discover that they have an allergy to nightshade vegetables, which makes their tongue swell up and causes breathing difficulties. They sue you, and you have to defend yourself, whether you are guilty or innocent. Defence costs a fortune.

People who are allergic to nightshade vegetables generally know this already, but these examples illustrate a point. You just can't be too careful. Dr Atkins who created the Atkins diet was sued a couple of times, over the adverse effects of his diet. Lots of people who work in the field of health get sued, and it makes sense to have insurance.

In Western culture, broadly speaking, people agree with the medical profession, and going against medical advice is ill-advised. Few people would argue that Western society needs to consume more fruit and vegetables – the government promotes it. So I tend to focus on the things that everybody agrees on.

Things that are undisputed are easier to sell for one thing. But they are also less controversial and less likely to get you into trouble, than some of the more radical ideas in the area of natural health.

I have been known to suggest cutting down on junk foods, or eliminating wheat or dairy from your diet for a week or two, to see if a problem then resolves itself. This borders on controversial. Personally I'm uncomfortable going very much further than this, without knowing the readers' backgrounds. So I try to keep my health writing fairly conventional – and to be honest, that's what people want anyway. They don't want to hear about our toxic world and what they shouldn't do. They are much more interested in being told to eat more apples and take a relaxing bath, than to eliminate cakes from their diet and avoid chemical toxins in their home.

Photographic permissions

It's worth being aware that when you take photographs on private land, you should at least in theory, have permission from the landowner if you intend to use the photographs commercially. In practice, implicit permission is usually assumed unless photography is explicitly forbidden.

Visitor attractions that invite people onto their land usually make it clear if photography is forbidden – sometimes it specifically says that commercial photography is forbidden on your entrance ticket. Hatfield House in Hertfordshire explicitly forbids commercial photography on their land, as do the Harry Potter Studios in Watford. Check the terms shown on your ticket, also check the terms on their website, and if in doubt, check with the press office, or request special permissions for your project. They are usually very obliging.

If you're using a model in your photographs, you'll need to have a model release form which permits you to use the photographs commercially – it ensures that the contract between the photographer and the model is completely clear and legally binding, and it requires the model to have some kind of 'valuable consideration' for his or her work.

Publishing a photo of a child who is subject to child protection measures can be a criminal offence, so it makes sense to ensure that you always have written permission from parents or guardians to publish any photographs of children. If a child walks into one of my photographs, I usually just wait until they are facing away, so that the child in my shot cannot be identified.

Exercise

Consider the risk of libel in your profession. Write down any work that you've done to date. Is there anything that has the potential to offend anyone? If in doubt, or even if you think there's a risk, get a quote for writer's insurance and just consider your options. Don't dismiss insurance without giving the risks due consideration and weighing up the cost of insurance against the risks of losing your home while defending yourself in a copyright or libel case.

Chapter 22

For struggling new writers – overcoming negativity

Many new writers struggle to get started and it's often not helped by the negativity of other people. Are you a writer who is surrounded by a supportive family and people who believe in you? Or are you – like so many have been at one time or another – in a position where you face daily criticism, antagonism and disrespect for following your writing dreams?

I didn't find it easy trying to get started when I was a teenager, but there are ways of managing the situation if you find yourself surrounded by rejection letters and negativity.

1) Understand the bigger picture

Most people think a comfortable lifestyle is one where you can support yourself and don't have to worry too much about paying the bills. So when you say you want to enter a profession with no guaranteed income, erratic payment schedules, and periods without work, it's only natural that a few people might question it. Maybe they are just looking out for your best interests.

However, there is nothing as fulfilling as doing a job you enjoy. It easily makes up for a shortfall in salary. The real challenge is whether you can convince those around you that your modest income, while you try to get established, will be sufficient to meet your outgoings.

If convincing your family is an impossible task, and you're not in a position to just try it and see, then trying to build up a regular part-time income from your writing makes sense. This might be exhausting and frustrating if you're working full-time in another job, but some people will never be convinced that you'll succeed until you prove them wrong.

The blogger Kris Heap, recently posted on www.successify .net, an inspirational message about ignoring your critics. Here's what he said: "The moment you decide to believe in something worthwhile you will come up against some critics. Every worthy cause comes with criticism from those too timid to try it themselves. In fact, if you never meet with any criticism, you may want to set higher goals for yourself! Critics are those insecure people who have never dared to invest themselves in a great cause or dream. They cannot accept the fact that someone will do the things that they are afraid to try themselves, so they put all of their energy into criticising people. They want everyone to be like them so that they can feel okay about themselves."

When I asked Kris permission to quote from his blog in this book, he said yes, and added, "I think my family felt I was wasting my time for the first little while. But eventually I started getting emails from people all over the world to thank me for inspiring them to achieve more. Sometimes family and friends just don't catch the vision of what we are doing."

Don't let critics quash your dreams, but do get a sense of balance and try to understand the bigger picture – perhaps some of your critics really do want job security for you, and have your best interests at heart. That's not to say they're right of course, but sometimes a willingness to compromise can make life easier at home.

2) Seek out positive influences

Build up a network of contacts who are supportive of your ambitions. For example, join a writers' group and attend writers' conferences. These activities provide opportunities for you to mix with like-minded people. Go online and join writers' forums where you can share ideas and experiences.

Meeting other people in the same boat can give you a sense of community and belonging, and you'll often encourage one another in your ambitions, share tips and help each other to hone your literary skills. You might even discover new genres that you're interested in exploring and you'll probably develop wider interests in literature as well as have your eyes opened to new opportunities in writing that you hadn't considered before.

3) Show off your successes

Generate respect for your work by showcasing your successes. Writers' talents are often overlooked until they become well known, but an impressive portfolio can go a long way to generating more work, as well as convincing your family and friends that this is a serious occupation for you. A website displaying your successes is a great place to start.

If you haven't had much success to date, why not try different styles, types of writing and genres? It might be that your greatest talents lie in writing about gardening, rather than writing novels. Perhaps that's why you're reading this book!

Blow your own trumpet and take articles that you've had published round to show people. Don't be modest about your successes. Show people how good you are and this will help to earn respect for your writing as a serious occupation, whether it's full-time or part-time.

4) Avoid interruptions

As a writer, it's ever so easy to get distracted with other tasks and responsibilities, but it's important, if you want to really make a success of it, that you manage your time effectively. It's a good idea to work to regular hours, say 8am until 5pm if you're embarking on a new writing career full-time.

You also need to be firm with people who call throughout the day thinking you have time on your hands to run errands. Explain that you are working to deadlines – you have a lot on. Or that you need to generate X amount of work, or send five proposals, before you can stop for a breather. But also remember, everyone needs a break from time to time. I personally enjoy a short walk every day to stretch my legs and get fresh air into my lungs. Get the balance right but don't allow people to take advantage of the fact that you're not tied to an office.

5) Be true to yourself and your dreams

Whether you're writing full-time or part-time, don't let rejection or others people's lack of vision, stop you from following your dreams. If your publishing ambitions are not taking off, all is not lost. With the growth in e-books and the popularity of e-readers, it's much cheaper and easier now than ever in the past, to bring your book to market without a publisher.

If you enjoy writing for pleasure but can't find a publisher, you can sell e-books, or just start a blog and let people enjoy your work for free.

You don't have to be earning a living as a writer to feel liberated as a published writer and be appreciated by your readership, even if that readership is modest in the beginning.

Besides, what begins as an unpaid blog, can develop as a solid fan base and regular readership, who are interested in your work. This in turn, often leads to bigger and better things.

6) Write under the radar

If you're living with people who don't support or respect your writing, then it may be less antagonistic to keep a low profile where your writing is concerned. That doesn't mean writing in secret, but keeping discussions about writing to the confines of your writers' group might help.

Enjoy writing as a hobby but don't discuss your ambitions with your family if the feedback is likely to be critical, disappointing or demoralising – just share your successes. If you become so successful that you are able to make the leap to full-time writer, then the evidence of this will be clear. Until then, it might be better to quietly keep a low profile and write under the radar.

7) Write for pleasure

Most well-known writers had a hard time getting started. Try not to let rejection get you down. Enjoy writing for the pleasure it gives you. Anything else is a bonus!

8) Don't be discouraged – everything's competitive!

A recent episode of Britain's Got Talent showed singer, Jordan O'Keefe, take the stage with his guitar and wow the judges, making it into the finals. He studied music at university – no thanks to his dad, who went to the university and changed his course to business. A heated argument ensued, as you can imagine.

Jordan switched his course back to music, and when he went to audition for Britain's Got Talent, industry guru, Simon Cowell, said he had a bright future in the music industry. Jordan's dad swallowed his pride, apologised for trying to block Jordan's aspirations, and came to watch him perform in the semi-finals.

Jordan's second performance received an excellent critique too, winning him a place in the finals.

Actress and singer, Amanda Holden, who was on the judging panel, said Jordan was right to follow his dreams, adding that in the downbeat economic climate, everything is competitive. Almost every job attracts dozens of applicants so you might as well aim high and do what you most want to do.

This comment reminded me of a conversation I'd had with my own dad, two years earlier. In 2011, at the launch of my full-time writing career, he argued that the industry was too competitive and said I wouldn't make it – an argument he's been perpetuating for the past 25 years. All grown up, I wasn't going to listen to his unfounded negativity any more.

"Trying to get a job in marketing management is competitive!" I argued, "Anything decent is competitive!" And it's true. Almost everything is competitive – even the low paid jobs that you might think are undesirable, are competitive.

Thinking back to the 1990s recession, when I first seriously had aspirations to follow a career in writing, I couldn't get a job in McDonalds. I was turned down for a position stacking supermarket shelves and rejected for a number of jobs in care.

I had good grades in English and writing was my only real strength, but I couldn't get a staff position at a newspaper either, and dad, who called the shots at the time, didn't consider freelance writing a suitable career choice.

However, as an adult, when you're living independently there is something to be said for doing what you're good at and embracing what you're passionate about – even if it's a bit unconventional and doesn't meet with everyone's approval!

Despite what other people think, the employment environment is incredibly competitive whatever field of work you choose – especially at times of economic recession.

I don't agree with Amanda Holden on many things, but I'd agree that it makes sense to monetise your greatest talents, especially during times of economic recession. After all, if you can't make money doing what you're good at, what hope do you have trying to fit into a more conventional role, for which you have no natural spark? Reach for your dreams and show off your talents. In the modern working environment, almost *everything worthwhile* is competitive. *Enjoyable* work is competitive. *Fulfilling* work is competitive.

Negative people will always say you'll fail, but have self-belief, then get out there and compete. If you're any good, and you don't give up, you'll probably succeed eventually.

9) Manage your expectations

While it's good to follow your dreams, I wouldn't advocate giving up the day job until you have pretty reassuring signs of success. I took redundancy because the offer was good and the alternative looked bleak. I didn't take redundancy specifically to build a career as a writer.

For the early months of my new-launched writing career, I

was applying for marketing jobs alongside my writing activities (increasingly sporadically as my freelance work grew and time passed). But I had good evidence of success before I completely stopped applying for external employment in what some might call, 'a proper job'.

Even then, for the first year, I did a bit of gardening, cleaning, laundry, and typing to bring in more funds and to help justify my existence as a freelance writer. My first year's takings were considerably less than the minimum wage, despite working long hours seven days a week, and being completely dedicated to my craft.

You are unlikely to see instant success and a salary to match. Building up your freelance writing business takes time and huge determination. Don't quit the day job and expect it to fall into your lap. It might be that you're better suited to a part-time writing career.

I was lucky to have the complete support of my husband, who was willing to pay the bills while I worked to build up my writing work from scratch. I started with no contacts and little experience. It was the time spent in those early days, pitching all day long, to try and win commissions in freelance writing, that got me up and running quickly.

The bottom line is only go full-time when finances and circumstances allow you to succeed or to fail without dismal consequences. If, in the event of failure, you stand to lose your house, I just wouldn't risk it.

10) Remember the hardships of great writers

- William Wordsworth was ridiculed for many years before he was recognised as a great poet.
- Stephen King had his early works rejected by publishers.
- Thomas Hardy burnt his first novel because he couldn't find anyone to publish it.

- James Herbert had 6 publishers reject his first best-selling novel. The seventh publisher accepted it, and he spent the rest of his life as Britain's best-selling horror writer.

Exercise

Write down your greatest challenges as a writer and think about how you can overcome them. What can you change to make your writing journey a more pleasurable experience?

Chapter 23

Focus on productivity

As I begin this chapter, it's early on a Saturday morning at the start of a bank holiday weekend. I am going to Basildon Park today to cover the house and gardens which were used in the 2005 film, Pride and Prejudice. Then tomorrow I'm off to Highclere Castle to cover a piece on Downton Abbey. On Monday, I'm going to West Wycombe Park to see where Austenland was filmed.

Each of these glorious stately homes has impressive gardens which I cover for a variety of magazines. But you'll notice that I don't stop working just because it's a weekend. Although it's Saturday, I was up at 7am and I've already proofread an interview with a blind man for a woman's weekly, and sought permission to quote Kris Heap from Successify in this book!

Writing is my life, and my husband comes along for the ride, visiting film locations and helping with the photography. I try to achieve something every day, moving my writing ahead a little bit further, even if it's just a small amount of progress. I do take breaks and reduce the workload at weekends though. I benefit from a break and don't want to burn out, or take too much time away from my good relationship with my husband.

During the week, it can be easy to spend too much time on social media, doing the washing, or tidying the house. While it can be beneficial to move about physically, catch up with friends online, and get away from your writing desk for a while, it is helpful to set targets for your productivity, and to be aware if you are spending too much time on tasks that are unproductive to your writing agenda.

Even cooking is a justifiable productive activity when you're writing recipes for foodie magazines, so it's certainly not necessary to be tied to your desk all day, but you'll feel more satisfied with your writing achievements, if at the end of each day you've achieved a good draft, submitted an article, written 1000 words on your book, or enjoyed a day out which will serve as the basis for an article later in the week.

Some people try to write 1000 words each day. It's a very good discipline. These words don't need to be perfect, but getting a draft down, can be very satisfying, even if it takes two days of tidying and editing to perfect it afterwards! I find submitting articles is rewarding... but only if you're sure they're as good as they can be, and don't have a flurry of anxiety afterwards because you didn't spend enough time perfecting it!

Ways to increase your productivity include:

- setting a target word count that you hope to achieve on a daily or weekly basis;
- limiting your social media time to once in the morning and once in the afternoon;
- only tidying the house in the evenings (you wouldn't normally spend your working day tidying up the house, so why do it when you're self-employed?);
- if you need to get out for a walk or a break, use the time to generate ideas;
- manage other people's expectations on your time so that they are not constantly imposing on your writing time, to the detriment of your productivity.

Exercise

Set targets for the amount of work you want to achieve in any given week, by word count, assignments commissioned, essential visits and photography. Do you fall short of these targets at the moment? Think about how you can improve your productivity and commit to doing one thing better next week.

Chapter 24

End game: how writing for a living has changed my life

I always loved books and wanted to write for a living, but various things prevented me doing so until my late 30s, when my career in marketing ended in redundancy. It took a leap of faith in my ability and with a huge amount of effort and determination, but today I have made it as a freelance journalist. I now write regularly for food, health and gardening magazines, and women's weeklies.

What I didn't expect after I took redundancy and launched my new career, was to learn so much about myself and about the world around me!

I have learnt about the kings and queens of England – perhaps something you'd think I learnt at school, but it didn't sink in at school. I've learnt about different religions and spiritual groups. I've learnt a lot about the way people lived in Victorian times, and about the Second World War. It's been an incredible learning journey – doing interviews and research for stories. I find history really interesting and wonder how I managed to be so disinterested at school! I've learnt about beekeeping, environmental issues, photography and gardening.

On a more personal level, I have discovered that I am rubbish at writing conflict fiction because I don't know how to respond in conflict situations. It's actually a real problem in developing my fiction portfolio because most fiction thrives on conflict!

In real life I've never been able to cope with conflict: whether it came in the guise of bullies, critical parents, or conflicts at work! I grew up with ambitions to become a hermit – something I've pretty much achieved now. Working at home, alone in my study, all I have to do is produce good work. No one cares how I do it. There is no conflict and no one makes life difficult.

I am incredibly driven and tenacious, taking editors' rejections on the chin and going back for more! This drive has helped me to increase my writing workload, despite a difficult economy and a shrinking market for conventionally published material. My tenacity has been destructive in the past, but now having the opportunity to channel my passion and determination into constructive things, I am much more fulfilled as a person. Writing for a living has opened my eyes to so many things that I never took an interest in before. Suddenly I find myself speaking to elderly people about their wartime experiences, seeking heritage attractions on my holidays, and going to the local photography club to learn how to improve my photography skills. I am still working towards achieving photographs with a real 'wow' factor to accompany my articles.

Becoming a full-time professional writer has brought dramatic change to my life, challenged my outlook, created new interests, and developed new skills. But most of all, it has helped me to discover the 'real me'. For years I felt crushed by other people's expectations about how I should look and behave, what I should think, where I should work, and what ambitions I should have (and not have).

"A square peg in a round hole" is how my mum used to put it, as I strived to meet other people's expectations of me and almost invariably failed. But finally, being a freelance writer allows me to just be myself. No conflict, no criticism, just steady work doing what I've always been good at – writing.

Chapter 25

Research and resources

This chapter is a collection of useful resources for writers, to help with finding work, training, conferences, or simply for inspiration!

Some of these opportunities are UK based (.co.uk), and others are worldwide (.com). They are a selection of the opportunities and are not definitive. Search more widely for more options in your own locality.

Writers' Handbooks
The Writers' and Artists' Yearbook in the UK:
   www.writersandartists.co.uk
The Australian Writer's Marketplace:
   www.awmonline.com.au
The Writers Market in the USA:
   www.writersmarket.com

Online job boards for writers
www.elance.com
www.guru.com
www.jobs.guardian.co.uk/jobs/media/journalism
www.journalism.co.uk
www.holdthefrontpage.co.uk
www.gorkanajobs.co.uk/jobs/journalist
www.indeed.co.uk/Journalism-jobs

Journalism courses
www.nctj.com
www.guardian.co.uk/guardian-masterclasses/about-masterclasses
www.journalism.co.uk/vocational-skills-study/s43

www.bjtc.org.uk
www.city.ac.uk/arts-social-sciences/journalism/city-journalism-
courses
www.sheffield.ac.uk/journalism
www.writersbureau.com

Writers' groups

Don't be a lonely writer. Writers' groups can provide feedback
and support that make you feel part of a community, and help
you to make new friends. They can egg you on, help you grow as
a writer, and give you confidence. This is particularly helpful if
others around you fail to understand what writing means to you,
and are dismissive of your writing ambitions. Search online for a
writers' group in your local area. I am a member of Chiltern
Writers: www.chilternwriters.org

Online communities for writers

www.writerscafe.org
www.writers-online.co.uk
www.scribophile.com
www.greatwriting.co.uk
www.writers-network.com
www.youngwritersonline.net
www.completelynovel.com
www.linkedin.com/groups
www.facebook.com/groups/the.writers.bureau
www.facebook.com/groups/ukpress
www.writelink.co.uk

Membership associations

National Union of Journalists:
www.nuj.org.uk
Society of Authors:
www.societyofauthors.net

Author's Guild USA:
www.authorsguild.org
National Writers' Union USA:
www.nwu.org
The American Society of Journalists and Authors:
www.asja.org

Websites for hooks and inspiration

Latest science news:
www.sciencedaily.com
Big dates in British history:
www.information-britain.co.uk/famousdates.php
What happened in history on any given day:
www.datesinhistory.com
Holidays around the world:
www.earthcalendar.net
Bank holidays, and other notable dates:
www.bankholidaydates.co.uk

Professional indemnity insurance

www.imaginsurance.co.uk/writers.html
www.towergateprofessionalrisks.co.uk

Other useful websites

www.absolutewrite.com
www.goodreads.com
www.writerunboxed.com
www.worldwidefreelance.com
www.successify.net
http://royal.pingdom.com/2013/01/16/internet-2012-in-numbers

Publishers and Agents

MacMillan New Writing
www.panmacmillan.com/imprints

Authonomy:

www.authonomy.com

Find a Literary Agent:

www.literaryagent.co.uk

Writers' and Artists' Yearbook:

www.writersandartists.co.uk

Self-publishing

www.lulu.com

www.smashwords.com

www.lightningsource.com

https://kdp.amazon.com/self-publishing/signin

Blogging Sites

www.blogspot.com

www.wordpress.org

Conferences

www.writersconference.co.uk

www.southernwriters.co.uk

www.greatwriting.org.uk

www.writersworkshop.co.uk/events.html

www.newpages.com/writing-conferences

www.pwcwriters.org

Follow Susie Kearley on Social Media

Facebook:

www.facebook.com/susie.kearley.writer

Twitter:

www.twitter.com/susiekearley

**COMPASS
BOOKS**

Compass Books focuses on practical and informative 'how-to' books for writers. Written by experienced authors who also have extensive experience of tutoring at the most popular creative writing workshops, the books offer an insight into the more specialised niches of the publishing game.

In 2011 Susie Kearley quit a 15 year marketing career to start up as a freelance writer in the middle of a recession. In this book, she shares how, in under two years, she went from being an aspirational rookie, to working for some of the biggest names in publishing.

Susie explains how:

- she built up valuable contacts from nothing;
- she used her nutrition qualifications and background in natural health to spur her career forward;
- she generated numerous feature ideas from single opportunities;
- she sold articles on health, food and gardening topics to diverse and unexpected markets;
- her unrelenting perseverance and tenacity came good in the end, despite numerous obstacles;
- she challenged those who said she would never succeed and proved them wrong.

....

This book is inspirational. It provides valuable tips to get you started in writing for the health, food and gardening markets, and has wider relevance to other fields of journalism.

Interviews with other writers – all working in the health, food and gardening markets – give superb insight into the highlights and challenges that each of them have faced in this field of work. The book features interviews with some well-known writers and with others who are still building their reputation, including:

- **Amanda Hamilton**, celebrity nutritionist and health writer;
- **Jackie Lynch**, nutritionist and health writer;
- **Nick Baines**, travel writer focusing on food topics;
- **Sue Ashworth**, food and cookery writer;
- **John Negus**, gardening writer;
- **Helen Riches**, garden designer and writer.

Each of these professionals offers their own hints for getting published in their specialist markets.

Susie provides humorous accounts of the obstacles she faced, as well as tips on how to write a winning pitch, how to market yourself as a writer, and how to avoid legal issues. She provides anecdotes and personal insights that many freelance writers will relate to, on topics from getting paid, to quashing the myths of freelance writing.

This book is a valuable resource for anyone wanting to be a successful freelance writer in the health, food, and gardening markets.

www.compass-books.net

COMPASS
BOOKS

Body, Mind & Spirit
UK £11.99
US $19.95

US $19.95
ISBN 978-1-78279-304-5

Cover image © Shutterstock
Cover design by Design Deluxe

9 781782 793045